# CANDIDA CLEANSE DIET COOKBOOK FOR BEGINNERS



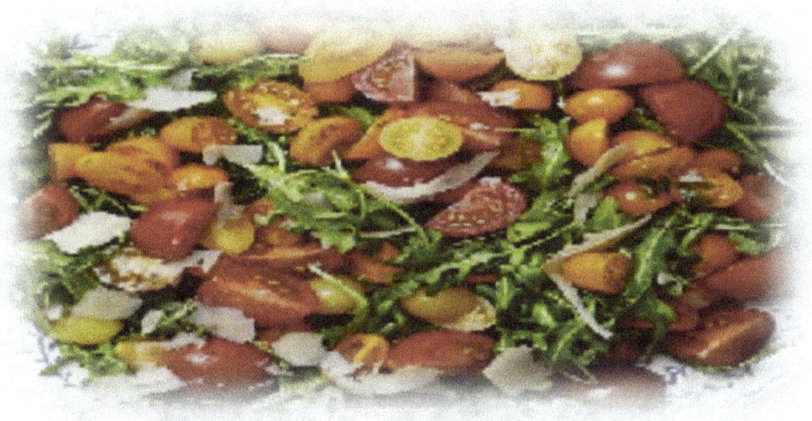

Unlock Your Health Potential with 55+ Delicious Anti-Fungal Recipes to Restore Your Gut and Achieve Optimal Wellness

*Dr. Laura Loeffler*

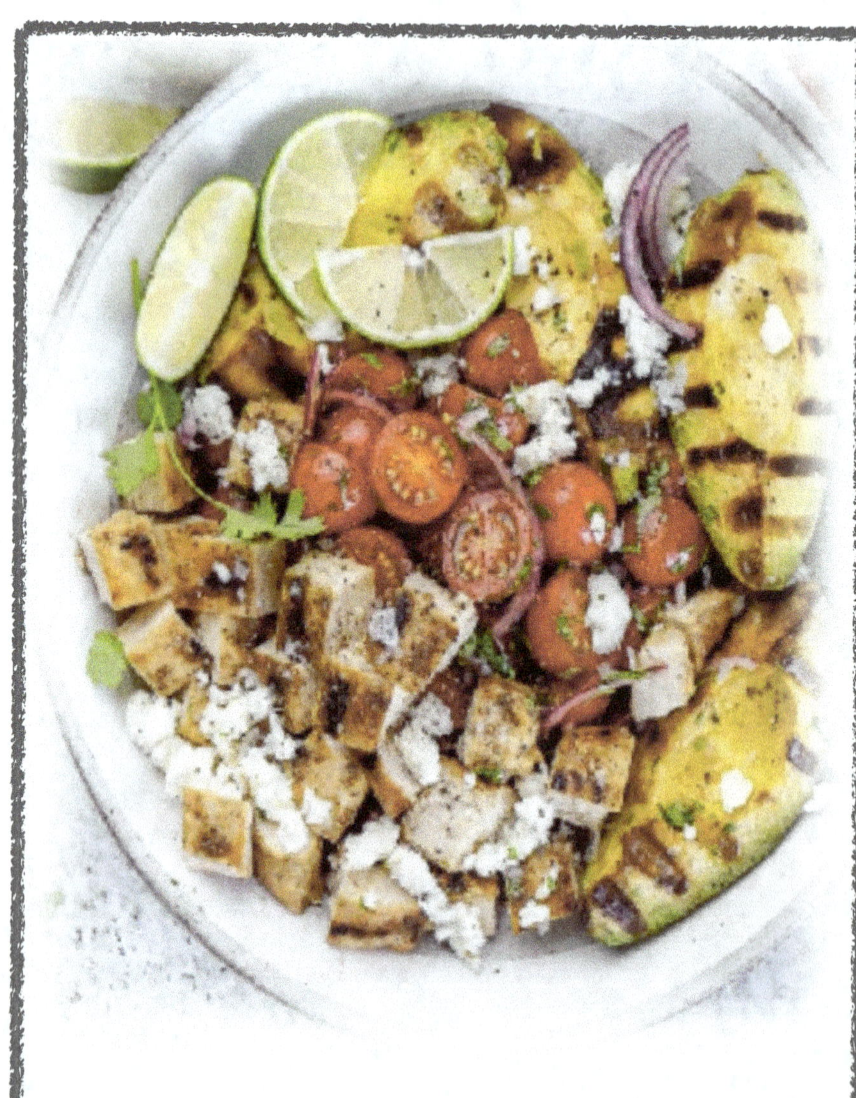

# Grilled Chicken Salad With Avocado

**SCAN THIS QR CODE TO GAIN ACCESS TO MORE OF MY BOOKS**

Dear Readers,

Thank you for opening this book. You've begun the process of reclaiming your health and becoming a more vibrant version of yourself. It's a path I've been on before, one marked by frustration, bewilderment, and, in the end, deep optimism.

In these pages, you'll find more than just recipes. You'll discover a battle strategy for your gut and a road map to navigating the maze of Candida overgrowth. You'll learn about the power of nutritious food, the silent orchestra of your microbiome, and the transforming potential that is within your grasp.

But know this: you are not alone. I've walked this path, experienced the highs and lows, and come out stronger on the other side. Now I'll share my experience, expertise, and kitchen with you.

Allow these dishes to be your cooking partners and guides on your journey. Enjoy the blast of flavor in a sun-drenched salad, the soothing warmth of a healthy soup, and the pleasure of a protein meal that fills your body and soul.

Remember, this is more than simply a cleansing; it is a paradigm change. It's about listening to your body, respecting its demands, and developing its full potential. It's about regaining your health and enjoying the full life that lies ahead.

So, thank you again for joining me. Let's cook, heal, and thrive together.

With warm wishes,

Dr. Laura Loeffler

# TABLE OF CONTENTS

# INTRODUCTION

Imagine a small renter living rent-free in your stomach. Candida albicans, a form of yeast, is often a tranquil resident that aids digestion and nutritional absorption. However, this nice roommate occasionally hosts a raucous party, bringing its fungal cousins and transforming your stomach into a chaotic nightclub. Candida overgrowth can have serious consequences for your health.

What causes this unwelcome growth? Imagine Candida as a sugar fiend. If you eat too much sugar, processed foods, and refined carbohydrates, you're essentially inviting a Candida invasion. Stress and medications can also upset the delicate balance of intestinal flora, giving Candida an unfair edge in the microbial mosh pit.

Candida overgrowth parties can have far-reaching repercussions. Common digestive symptoms include bloating, gas, and diarrhea. However, Candida's tentacles can extend well beyond the stomach, producing brain fog, lethargy, intractable skin conditions such as dermatitis, and even mood swings.

Years ago, I unwittingly hosted a roaring Candida festival. I suffered from unexplained lethargy, mental fog, and recurrent skin issues. Conventional medication provided little help, leaving me confused and dissatisfied. Then I discovered the realm of Candida cleanses, and it was like a beam of sunlight breaking through the gloom.

The Candida detox entails more than just avoiding sugary foods. It's about knowing your gut's complex ecosystem, which is filled with bacteria, both healthy and harmful. The cleanse seeks to restore balance by removing Candida's preferred foods (sugars and refined carbohydrates) while replenishing the beneficial bacteria with gut-friendly veggies, healthy fats, and fermented foods. It's a reset button for your stomach, an opportunity to evict unwelcome partygoers and create a healthy refuge.

Imagine navigating this nutritional change without a map. That is where the "Candida Cleanse Diet Cookbook for Beginners" comes in. It's your culinary compass, leading you through the maze of limitations with tasty, easy-to-follow recipes. Consider colorful salads, rich soups that warm your spirit, and protein meals that leave you feeling rejuvenated. But these aren't just any dishes; they're Candida-friendly, full of taste, and a gut-loving delight.

Understanding and managing the Candida cleanse diet entails more than simply following a list of guidelines on your plate. It's about going on a path of self-discovery, learning to listen to your body's cues, and gaining control over your health.

It's about tending the delicate garden within you, creating an atmosphere in which the good guys thrive while the evil people are respectfully shown the door. With the appropriate supervision, a "Candida Cleanse Diet Cookbook for Beginners" may help you become a healthier, happier version of yourself. So put on your chef's hat, grab your cookbook, and prepare to nurture a gut garden full of bright health.

# CHAPTER 1

## *UNDERSTANDING, BENEFITS, AND PRACTICAL STEPS*

The Candida Cleanse Diet has gained popularity as an effective approach to treating Candida overgrowth, a disease caused by an imbalance of the yeast Candida in the body. This detailed book delves into what a Candida Cleanse Diet comprises, the multiple advantages it provides, methods for recognizing Candida overgrowth, and practical measures to prepare for and carry out a successful cleanse. It also discusses the importance of choosing the correct meals, avoiding possible triggers, and having the required kitchen supplies to maximize the Candida Cleanse experience.

## What Is the Candida Cleansing Diet?

The Candida Cleanse Diet is a dietary strategy that aims to restore the microbiota and reduce the overgrowth of Candida, a yeast that lives naturally in the human body. This diet focuses on removing Candida-promoting foods, such as refined sugars and processed carbs, while integrating anti-fungal and nutrient-dense alternatives. The goal is to establish an environment in the body that discourages Candida multiplication, resulting in improved gut health and overall well-being.

# Benefits of Candida Cleanse

1. **Gut Health and Digestive Harmony:**

   ✓ **Balancing the Microbiome:** The Candida Cleanse helps restore a healthy balance of gut bacteria, promoting optimal digestion and nutrient absorption.

   ✓ **Alleviating Digestive Discomfort:** By reducing Candida overgrowth, individuals may experience relief from bloating, gas, and other digestive issues.

2. **Enhanced Immune Function:**

   ✓ **Strengthening the Immune System:** A balanced microbiome positively impacts the immune system, reducing susceptibility to infections and illnesses.

   ✓ **Reducing Chronic Inflammation:** Candida overgrowth is linked to chronic inflammation, and the cleanse helps alleviate this burden on the immune system.

3. **Increased energy and mental clarity:**

   ✓ **Mitigating Fatigue:** By addressing the factors contributing to Candida overgrowth, individuals often report increased energy levels and reduced fatigue.

   ✓ **Addressing Brain Fog:** Improved gut health is associated with better cognitive function, alleviating symptoms like brain fog, and improving mental clarity.

4. **Skin Health and Radiance:**

   ✓ **<u>Minimizing Skin Infections:</u>** Candida overgrowth can manifest in skin issues; the cleanse may lead to clearer skin by reducing yeast-related infections.

   ✓ **<u>Promoting a Healthy Complexion:</u>** A balanced diet and reduced inflammation contribute to a healthier complexion.

5. **Weight Management:**

   ✓ **<u>Supporting Weight Loss:</u>** A Candida Cleanse often involves eliminating processed and sugary foods, contributing to weight loss.

   ✓ **<u>Regulating Metabolism:</u>** A balanced gut microbiome supports metabolic functions, aiding in weight management.

# How To Know if You Have Candida Overgrowth

1. **Recognizing Common Symptoms:**

   ✓ **<u>Digestive Issues:</u>** Persistent bloating, gas, and irregular bowel movements may indicate Candida overgrowth.

   ✓ **<u>Fatigue and Weakness:</u>** Chronic fatigue, low energy levels, and muscle weakness are common signs.

   ✓ **<u>Skin Problems:</u>** Recurrent skin infections, rashes, or persistent acne may be linked to Candida.

✓ **<u>Mood Swings and Mental Health Concerns:</u>** Anxiety, depression, and mood swings can be associated with an imbalance in the gut flora.

2. **Diagnostic tests and consultation:**

✓ **<u>Candida Overgrowth Tests:</u>** Various tests, including blood tests and stool analyses, can help diagnose Candida overgrowth.

✓ **<u>Seeking Professional Guidance:</u>** Consultation with a healthcare professional is crucial for accurate diagnosis and personalized treatment plans.

# Preparing for the Cleanse

1. **Mental and emotional preparation:**

✓ **<u>Setting Realistic Goals:</u>** Establish achievable goals for the cleanse to avoid frustration and maintain motivation.

✓ **<u>Understanding the Cleanse Process:</u>** Educate yourself about what to expect during the cleanse, both physically and emotionally.

2. **Gradual Dietary Transition:**

✓ **<u>Phasing Out Trigger Foods:</u>** Slowly reduce the intake of foods that promote Candida growth, such as sugars and processed carbohydrates.

✓ **<u>Introducing Candida-Fighting Foods</u>:** Gradually incorporate anti-fungal foods like garlic, coconut oil, and cruciferous vegetables.

3. **Lifestyle Adjustments:**

✓ **<u>Managing stress</u>:** Adopt stress management techniques, such as meditation or yoga, to support overall well-being.

✓ **<u>Incorporating Regular Exercise</u>:** Regular physical activity helps boost the immune system and aids in detoxification.

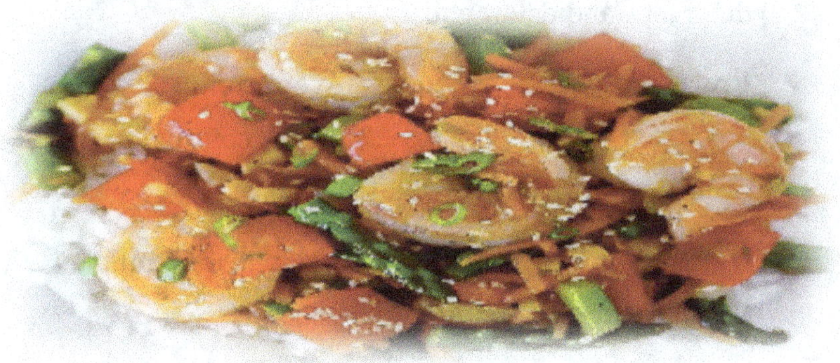

# Foods To Include and Avoid

1. **Candida-Friendly Foods:**

✓ **<u>Non-Starchy Vegetables</u>:** Broccoli, kale, spinach, and other non-starchy vegetables are rich in nutrients and support a healthy gut.

- ✓ **<u>Lean Proteins:</u>** Choose lean protein sources like poultry, fish, and plant-based proteins to maintain muscle health.

- ✓ **<u>Healthy Fats:</u>** Avocado, olive oil, and nuts provide essential fatty acids without promoting Candida growth.

- ✓ **<u>Probiotic-rich foods:</u>** Incorporate fermented foods like sauerkraut and yogurt with live cultures to promote a healthy balance of gut bacteria.

2. **Foods to avoid:**

- ✓ **<u>Refined Sugars:</u>** Eliminate sugary foods and beverages that fuel Candida growth.

- ✓ **<u>Processed Carbohydrates:</u>** Avoid refined grains and processed carbohydrates, as they contribute to yeast overgrowth.

- ✓ **<u>Dairy Products:</u>** Dairy can be a source of inflammation and may exacerbate Candida symptoms.

- ✓ **<u>Alcohol and caffeine:</u>** These substances can disrupt gut health and contribute to Candida overgrowth.

# Kitchen Essentials for Candida Cleanse

1. ***<u>Stocking a Candida-Friendly Pantry:</u>***

✓ **<u>Alternative Flours and Grains:</u>** Almond flour, coconut flour, and quinoa provide nutritious alternatives to traditional flours and grains.

✓ **<u>Natural Sweeteners:</u>** Stevia, monk fruit, or xylitol can replace refined sugars in recipes.

✓ **<u>Nut and Seed Butters:</u>** Healthy spreads like almond butter or sunflower seed butter add flavor and nutrients.

2. **Essential kitchen tools:**

✓ **<u>Blender and Food Processor:</u>** Essential for creating smoothies, sauces, and other Candida-friendly recipes.

✓ **<u>Fermentation Tools:</u>** Support the production of fermented foods like kimchi or sauerkraut, which promote a healthy gut.

✓ **<u>Quality Cookware:</u>** Non-toxic cookware ensures that your meals are free from harmful substances that may impact gut health.

3. **Meal Planning and Preparation:**

✓ **<u>Batch Cooking Strategies:</u>** Plan and prepare meals in batches to save time and ensure adherence to the Candida Cleanse.

✓ <u>**Creating Balanced and Varied Meals:**</u> Incorporate a variety of Candida-fighting foods to ensure a well-rounded and satisfying diet during the cleanse.

The Candida Cleanse Diet is an innovative journey to better health and vigor. Anyone may achieve holistic well-being by knowing the diet's principles, recognizing its advantages, spotting indicators of Candida overgrowth, and emotionally and practically preparing for the cleanse. Choosing the correct meals, avoiding possible triggers, and possessing the necessary kitchen gear all contribute to the cleanse's efficacy. By implementing these behaviors, people not only manage Candida overgrowth but also lay the groundwork for long-term health and fitness. This detailed book provides a road map for anybody looking to confidently and successfully complete the Candida Cleanse.

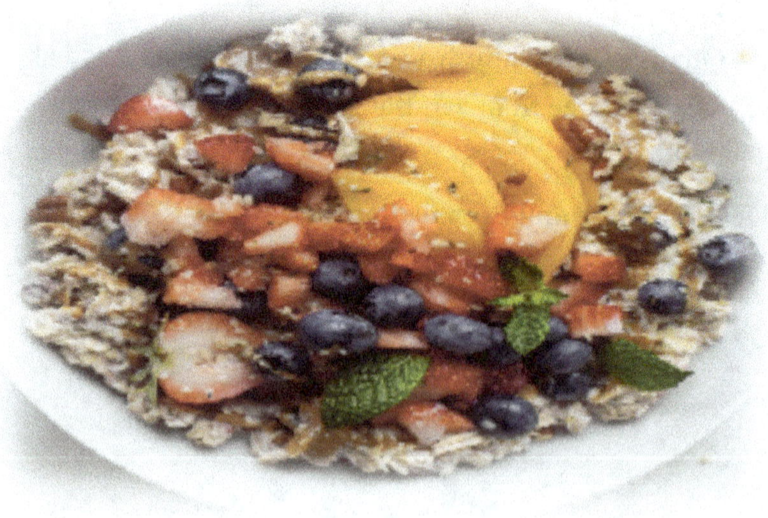

# CHAPTER 2

## CANDIDA-FRIENDLY BREAKFAST DELIGHT RECIPES

## Quick-And-Easy Avocado Mousse

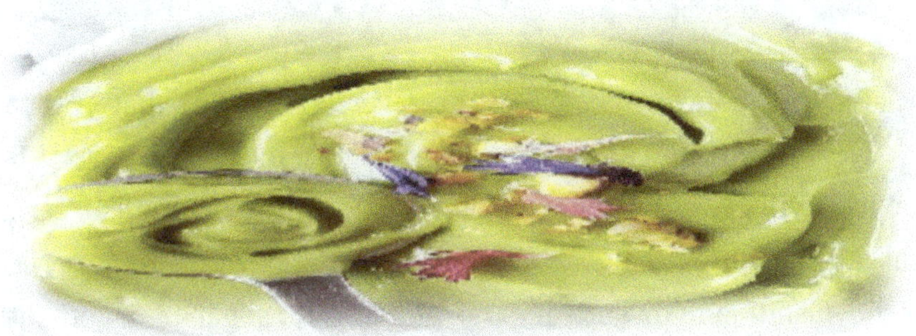

### *Ingredients:*

- ✓ 1 avocado, peeled and seeded
- ✓ 1/2 cup unsweetened plain yogurt
- ✓ 4 tablespoons canned full-fat coconut milk
- ✓ 2 tablespoons of fresh lime or lemon juice
- ✓ 1/4 cup mixed berries (optional)
- ✓ 1 tablespoon unsweetened coconut flakes (optional)

### *Preparation:*

4. In a blender or food processor, combine the avocado, yogurt, coconut milk, and lime or lemon juice. Blend until smooth and creamy.

5. Spoon the mousse into a serving dish or glass.

6. Top with mixed berries and unsweetened coconut flakes, if desired.

7. Serve right away or put it in the fridge until you're ready to eat.

Nutritional Value:

***Nutritional Value (per serving):*** Calories: 330, Fat: 29g, Carbohydrates: 16g, Fiber: 10g, Protein: 7g, Sugar: 3g, Sodium: 60mg.

***Prep Time:*** 5 minutes

**N**ote: This avocado mousse is a versatile recipe that you can eat for breakfast, as a midday snack, or even as a dessert! It's packed with healthy fats, protein, and a few complex carbs, making it a filling, balanced, and super-healthy meal that's perfect for the Candida diet. The recipe is gluten-free, sugar-free, and anti-inflammatory, making it suitable for those with Candida overgrowth.

# *Happy Gut Bowl*

***Ingredients:***

- ✓ 2 tablespoons of olive or coconut oil, separated
- ✓ 1/2 cup of broccoli florets
- ✓ 1/2 cup sliced zucchini
- ✓ Salt and pepper to taste
- ✓ 1 egg
- ✓ 1/2 cup cooked quinoa
- ✓ 1 cup of mixed greens

✓ 1/2 avocado, thinly sliced

✓ 2-3 Tbsp. sauerkraut

✓ 1 radish, grated

✓ 1 green onion, thinly sliced

✓ 1/4 cup olive oil

✓ 2 Tbsp. sauerkraut juice

✓ 1/2 tsp. onion powder

✓ 1/2 tsp. dried herbs

✓ Salt and pepper to taste

✓ Powdered stevia to taste

### *Preparation:*

1. Heat 1 tablespoon of oil in a pan over average heat.

2. Add the broccoli and zucchini, and cook until soft.

3. Add salt and pepper.

4. Transfer to a bowl and reserve.

5. In the same skillet, melt the remaining 1 tablespoon of oil.

6. Crack the egg into the skillet and cook to your desired doneness.

7. In a small bowl, whisk together the olive oil, sauerkraut juice, onion powder, dried herbs, salt, pepper, and powdered stevia to make the vinaigrette.

8. In a serving bowl, arrange the cooked quinoa, mixed greens, sautéed vegetables, and sliced avocado.

9. Top with the fried egg, sauerkraut, grated radish, and green onion.

10. Drizzle the sauerkraut vinaigrette over the bowl.

11. Serve and enjoy!

***Nutritional Value (per serving):*** Calories: 480, Fat: 38g, Carbohydrates: 28g, Fiber: 9g, Protein: 12g, Sugar: 3g, Sodium: 320mg

***Prep Time:*** 15 minutes

**N**ote: This Gut-Restoring Breakfast Bowl is a nutritious and balanced meal that supports gut health and is suitable for the Candida diet. It is rich in healthy fats, fiber, and essential nutrients, making it a perfect choice for those looking to restore their gut health.

# *Rhubarb Muffins*

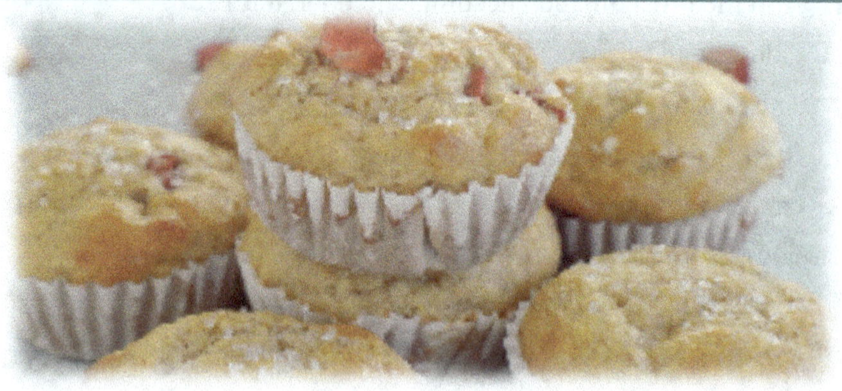

***Ingredients:***

- ✓ 1 cup of quinoa flour
- ✓ 1 cup light buckwheat flour
- ✓ 1 tsp. psyllium husk powder

✓ 1 tsp. cinnamon

✓ 1/2 tsp. salt

✓ 1 tsp. baking powder

✓ 1/2 tsp. baking soda

✓ 2 eggs

✓ 1/2 cup unsweetened plain yogurt

✓ 1/4 cup coconut oil

✓ 1/4 cup almond milk

✓ 1 tsp. vanilla extract

✓ Powdered stevia to taste

✓ 1 ½ cups rhubarb, sliced into half-inch pieces

**_Preparation:_**

1. Preheat the oven to 350 °F (175 °C).

2. Prepare a 12-cup muffin tin with paper liners.

3. In a large bowl, combine the quinoa flour, light buckwheat flour, psyllium husk powder, cinnamon, salt, baking powder, and baking soda. Whisk to combine, and set aside.

4. In another large bowl, whisk together the eggs, unsweetened plain yogurt, coconut oil, almond milk, vanilla extract, and powdered stevia.

5. Stir the wet and dry ingredients together until thoroughly blended.

6. Gently fold in the rhubarb chunks.

7. Divide the mixture evenly among the muffin cups you've prepared.

8. Bake for 20–25 minutes, or until a toothpick inserted into the middle of a muffin comes out clean.

9. Allow the muffins to cool in the pan for 5 minutes before transferring them to a wire rack to cool fully.

***Nutritional Value (per muffin):*** Calories: 180, Fat: 8g, Carbohydrates: 23g, Fiber: 4g, Protein: 5g, Sugar: 2g, Sodium: 220mg.

***Prep Time:*** 15 minutes

**N**ote: These rhubarb muffins are a delicious and nutritious breakfast option that is suitable for the Candida diet. They are gluten-free, sugar-free, and packed with protein, fiber, and healthy fats. If rhubarb is not available, you can substitute it with an equal amount of chopped strawberries for a similar flavor and texture.

## Savory Zucchini And Pesto Bread

***Ingredients:***

- ✓ 1 medium zucchini, grated
- ✓ 1 1/4 cups millet flour
- ✓ 3/4 cup blanched almond flour
- ✓ 1/2 cup light buckwheat flour
- ✓ 1 tablespoon psyllium husk powder
- ✓ 1/2 teaspoon salt
- ✓ 1 teaspoon baking soda
- ✓ 3 large eggs

- ✓  1/4 cup unsweetened almond milk
- ✓  1 tablespoon apple cider vinegar
- ✓  1/4 cup olive oil
- ✓  3 tablespoons of pesto

***Preparation:***

1. Preheat the oven to 350°F (175°C).
2. Put parchment paper inside and grease a 9-by-5-inch loaf pan.
3. In a large bowl, combine the grated zucchini, millet flour, almond flour, buckwheat flour, psyllium husk powder, salt, and baking soda.
4. In a separate bowl, whisk the eggs, almond milk, apple cider vinegar, and olive oil together.
5. Stir the wet and dry ingredients together until thoroughly blended.
6. Pour half of the batter into the loaf pan that was previously prepared.
7. Dot the batter with teaspoons of pesto, then swirl it in with a knife. Add the remaining batter on top.
8. Bake for 40–45 minutes, or until a toothpick put in the center comes out clean.
9. Allow the bread to cool in the pan for 10 minutes before transferring it to a wire rack to cool entirely.

***Nutritional Value (per serving):*** Calories: 220, Fat: 14g, Carbohydrates: 18g, Fiber: 3g, Protein: 7g, Sugar: 1g, Sodium: 280mg

**_Prep Time:_** 15 minutes

**N**ote: This savory zucchini and pesto bread is a delicious and nutritious breakfast option that is suitable for the Candida diet. It is gluten-free, sugar-free, and packed with protein, fiber, and healthy fats.

# Avocado-Baked Eggs With Vegetable Hash

## _Ingredients:_

- ✓  1/4 cup diced tomato
- ✓  1/4 cup diced zucchini
- ✓  1/4 cup diced yellow pepper
- ✓  1/4 cup diced onion
- ✓  2 Tbsp. olive oil, divided
- ✓  1 avocado, halved and seeded
- ✓  2 eggs, medium or large
- ✓  Salt and pepper to taste
- ✓  Fresh parsley, minced (optional)

## _Vegetable Hash Preparation:_

1.  Preheat the oven to 375°F (190°C).

2.  In a pan, heat 1 tablespoon of olive oil over average heat.

3.  Add the diced tomato, zucchini, yellow pepper, and onion.

4.  Sauté until the vegetables are tender and lightly browned. Season with salt and pepper.

5. Divide the vegetable hash evenly between the two avocado halves, filling the hollows where the seeds were removed.

**_Baked Eggs Preparation:_**

1. Crack an egg into each avocado half, on top of the vegetable hash.
2. Drizzle the remaining olive oil over the eggs and season with salt and pepper.
3. Place the avocado halves on a baking sheet and bake for 15 to 20 minutes, or until the egg whites are set and the yolks are starting to thicken.
4. Sprinkle with minced parsley, if desired.
5. Serve and enjoy!

**_Nutritional Value (per serving):_** Calories: 360 Fat: 32g, Carbohydrates: 14g, Fiber: 10g Protein: 10g Sugar: 2g Sodium: 150mg

**_Prep Time:_** 20 minutes

**N**ote: This Avocado Baked Eggs with Vegetable Hash recipe is a nutritious and balanced breakfast option that is suitable for the Candida diet. It is gluten-free, sugar-free, and packed with protein, fiber, and healthy fats.

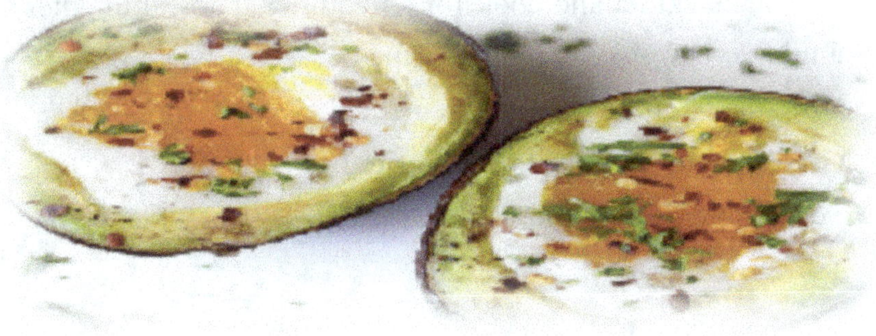

# *Smoky Rutabaga Hash*

## *Ingredients:*

- ✓ 1 large rutabaga, peeled and diced
- ✓ 1/2 cup diced onion
- ✓ 1/2 cup diced red bell pepper
- ✓ 2 tablespoons of olive oil
- ✓ 1 teaspoon smoked paprika
- ✓ 1/2 teaspoon garlic powder
- ✓ 1/2 teaspoon dried thyme
- ✓ Salt and pepper to taste
- ✓ Fresh parsley for garnish (optional)

## *Preparation:*

1. Heat the olive oil in a large pan over average heat.
2. Add the diced rutabaga, onion, and red bell pepper to the skillet. Sauté for 5 minutes.
3. Add the smoked paprika, garlic powder, dried thyme, salt, and pepper to the skillet. Stir to combine.
4. Cover the skillet and cook for an additional 15-20 minutes, or until the rutabaga is tender, stirring occasionally.
5. Once the rutabaga is tender, remove the skillet from the heat.
6. Garnish with fresh parsley, if desired.
7. Serve and enjoy!

<u>**Nutritional Value (per serving):**</u> Calories: 180, Fat: 9g, Carbohydrates: 24g, Fiber: 6g, Protein: 3g, Sugar: 10g, Sodium: 350mg.

<u>**Prep Time:**</u> 30 minutes

**N**<u>ote:</u> This Smoky Rutabaga Hash is a flavorful and nutritious breakfast option that is suitable for the Candida diet. It is gluten-free, sugar-free, and packed with fiber and essential nutrients.

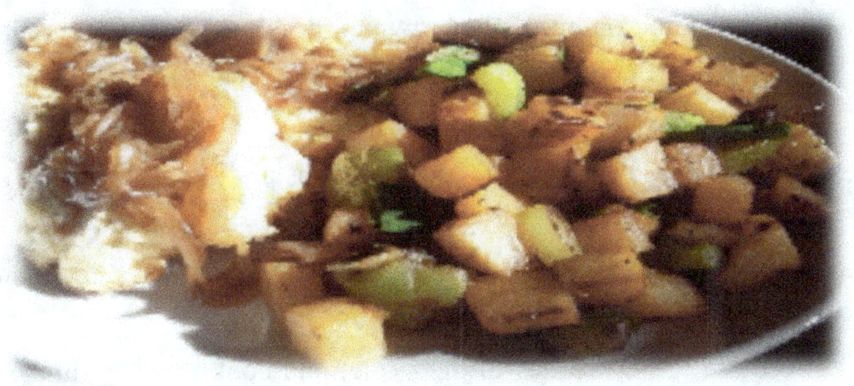

# Turkey and Sage Breakfast Patties

<u>**Ingredients:**</u>

✓ 1 lb. ground turkey

✓ 1 tablespoon finely minced fresh sage (or 1 teaspoon crumbled dry sage)

✓ 1 Tbsp green onions, finely minced

✓  1/2 tsp. dried thyme

✓  1/2 tsp. dried garlic flakes

✓  1/2 tsp salt

✓  1/4 tsp. pepper

✓  A pinch of red pepper flakes

✓  2 Tbsp. olive or coconut oil

### *Preparation:*

1. In a large bowl, combine the ground turkey, fresh sage (or dried sage), green onions, dried thyme, dried garlic flakes, salt, pepper, and a pinch of red pepper flakes. Mix until just combined.

2. Divide the mixture into 8 equal portions and shape each into a patty.

3. In a large skillet, heat the olive or coconut oil over medium heat.

4. Add the turkey patties to the skillet and cook for 4-5 minutes on each side, or until they are no longer pink in the center and the internal temperature reaches 165°F (74°C).

5. Once cooked, remove the patties from the skillet and place them on a plate lined with paper towels to drain any excess oil.

6. Serve the patties warmly, and enjoy!

Nutritional Value (per serving): Calories: 220, Fat: 15g, Carbohydrates: 1g, Protein: 20g, Sodium: 320mg.

***Prep Time:*** 20 minutes

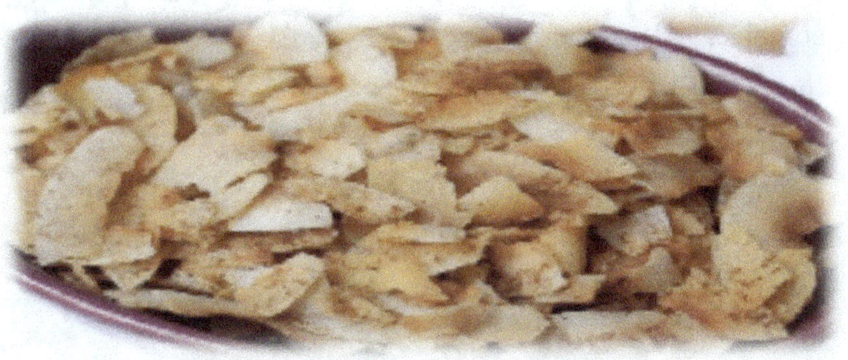

# *Cinnamon Coconut Crisp Cereal*

## *Ingredients:*

- ✓  1 1/2 cups almond flour
- ✓  1/2 cup unsweetened shredded coconut
- ✓  1 1/2 tsp. cinnamon
- ✓  1/4 tsp. salt
- ✓  1/4 tsp. baking soda
- ✓  1/2 teaspoon alcohol-free vanilla
- ✓  1/2 tsp. stevia powder
- ✓  1 Tbsp. coconut oil, melted
- ✓  1 egg white, at room temperature
- ✓  Blueberries (optional)

## **_Preparation:_**

1. Preheat the oven to 350°F (177°C).
2. In a medium bowl, combine almond flour, unsweetened shredded coconut, cinnamon, salt, and baking soda. Whisk to combine, and set aside.
3. In a small bowl, add alcohol-free vanilla, stevia powder, and melted coconut oil.
4. Whisk until the stevia powder has dissolved.
5. In a separate small dish, whisk the egg whites until foamy.
6. Combine the egg white and liquid mixture, and whisk thoroughly.
7. Add the liquid ingredients to the dry ingredients, and stir well to form a dough.
8. Roll out the dough between two sheets of parchment paper into a thin, 10 x 15-inch rectangle.
9. Transfer the cereal dough and parchment paper onto a baking sheet.
10. Remove the top sheet of parchment paper, and bake the dough for 12 minutes.
11. Transfer the cereal dough and parchment paper to a work surface.
12. With a sharp knife, carefully cut the dough into one-inch strips and then across into one-inch strips, creating one-inch squares.
13. Cool the cereal completely and serve with coconut or almond milk. Add blueberries if desired.

<u>**Nutritional Value (per serving):**</u> Calories: 180, Fat: 15g, Carbohydrates: 6g, Fiber: 3g, Protein: 7g, Sugar: 1g, Sodium: 150mg.

<u>**Prep Time:**</u> 30 minutes

**N**ote: This cinnamon-coconut crisp cereal is a delicious and nutritious breakfast option that is suitable for the Candida diet. It is gluten-free, sugar-free, and packed with protein, fiber, and healthy fats.

# Baked Eggs With Onions and Red Peppers

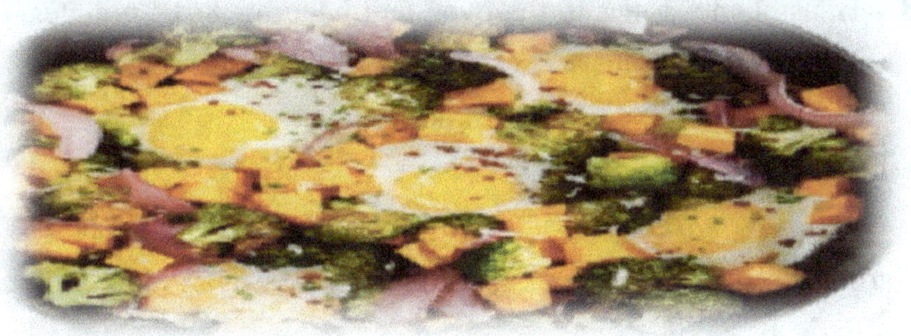

<u>**Ingredients:**</u>

- ✓ 1 Tbsp. olive oil
- ✓ 1/2 cup diced red bell pepper
- ✓ 1/2 cup diced onion
- ✓ 1/2 tsp. smoked paprika
- ✓ A pinch of red chili flakes
- ✓ 2 eggs

✓ Salt and pepper to taste

✓ Fresh parsley for garnish (optional)

### *Preparation:*

1. Preheat the oven to 375°F (190°C).

2. Heat the olive oil in a large oven-safe skillet on average heat.

3. In the skillet, combine the chopped red bell pepper and onion.

4. Simmer the veggies for 5 minutes or until they are tender.

5. Add the smoked paprika and red chili flakes to the skillet. Stir to combine.

6. Crack the eggs into the skillet, on top of the vegetables.

7. Season with salt and pepper, to taste.

8. Transfer the skillet to the oven and bake for 8–10 minutes, or until the egg whites are set and the yolks are still runny.

9. Garnish with fresh parsley, if desired.

10. Serve and enjoy!

***Nutritional Value (per serving):*** Calories: 180, Fat: 12g, Carbohydrates: 9g, Fiber: 2g, Protein: 9g, Sugar: 4g, Sodium: 150mg.

***Prep Time:*** 20 minutes

**N**ote: This baked egg skillet with red peppers and onions is a delicious and nutritious breakfast option that is suitable for the Candida diet. It is gluten-free, sugar-free, and packed with protein, fiber, and healthy fats.

# Bircher Muesli

<u>**Ingredients:**</u>

- ✓ 1½ cups unsweetened coconut flakes
- ✓ 1/2 cup of nuts like macadamias, hazelnuts, almonds, pecans, or walnuts
- ✓ 2 Tbsp. chia seeds
- ✓ 1½ cups unsweetened coconut milk
- ✓ Dash of alcohol-free vanilla (optional)
- ✓ 2 to 3 drops of liquid stevia (optional)
- ✓ 1/2 cup grated green apple (optional)
- ✓ Dash of nutmeg
- ✓ Pinch of salt

<u>**Preparation:**</u>

1. In a large bowl, combine the unsweetened coconut flakes, nuts, chia seeds, grated green apple (if using), nutmeg, and a pinch of salt. Mix well.
2. In a small bowl, combine the unsweetened coconut milk, alcohol-free vanilla (if using), and liquid stevia (if using). Stir well.
3. Pour the liquid mixture over the dry ingredients and stir until thoroughly incorporated.
4. Cover the bowl and refrigerate the muesli for at least 2 hours or overnight to let the flavors meld and the chia seeds soften.

5. Before serving, give the muesli a good stir and add a little extra coconut milk if it's too thick.

6. Serve the Bircher Muesli in individual bowls and top with a dollop of plain yogurt, if desired.

***Nutritional Value (per serving):*** Calories: 380, Fat: 34g, Carbohydrates: 14g, Fiber: 9g, Protein: 7g, Sugar: 4g, Sodium: 90mg.

***Prep Time:*** 10 minutes

**N**ote: This Bircher Muesli is a delicious and nutritious breakfast option that is suitable for the Candida diet. It is gluten-free, sugar-free, and packed with healthy fats, fiber, and essential nutrients.

# Southwestern Soufflé

***Ingredients:***

✓ 1 cup grilled or roasted chicken, cubed

✓ 1 cup avocado, cubed

✓ 1/4 cup roasted, peeled, seeded, and chopped green chilies

✓ 4 green onions, chopped

✓ 6 eggs

✓ 1/4 cup fresh cilantro, chopped

✓ 1/2 tsp salt

✓ 1/4 tsp. black pepper

✓ 1/4 tsp. chili powder

✓ 1/4 tsp. cumin

***Preparation:***

1. Preheat the oven to 350°F (175°C). Grease a 9-inch pie plate.
2. In a large bowl, combine the chicken, avocado, green chilies, green onions, and fresh cilantro.
3. In a separate bowl, beat the eggs, salt, black pepper, chili powder, and cumin.
4. Pour the egg mixture over the chicken and avocado mixture. Stir to combine.
5. Pour the mixture into the pie plate you've prepared.
6. Bake for 30-35 minutes, or until the eggs are firm and the top is golden brown.
7. Allow it to cool a few minutes before slicing and serving.

***Nutritional Value (per serving):*** Calories: 280, Fat: 20g, Carbohydrates: 6g, Fiber: 4g, Protein: 18g, Sugar: 1g, Sodium: 380mg.

***Prep Time:*** 15 minutes

**N**ote: This Southwestern Soufflé is a flavorful and protein-packed breakfast option that is suitable for the Candida diet. It is gluten-free, sugar-free, and rich in healthy fats and protein.

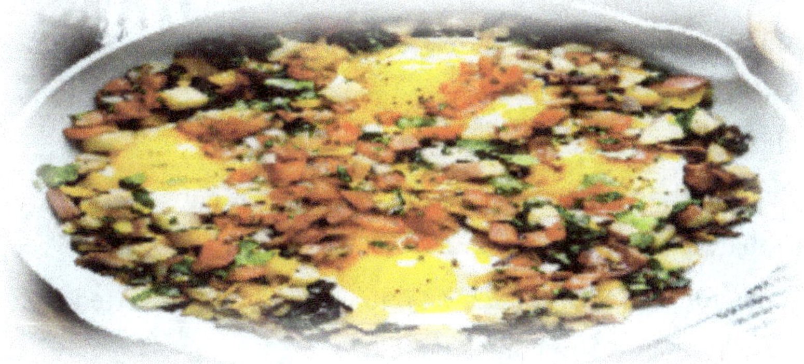

# Buckwheat Breakfast Muffins

**_Ingredients:_**

- ✓ 1 cup buckwheat flour
- ✓ 1/4 cup ground flaxseed
- ✓ 1 tsp. baking powder
- ✓ 1 tsp. cinnamon
- ✓ 1/4 tsp. salt
- ✓ 2 eggs
- ✓ 1 1/2 cups unsweetened almond milk
- ✓ 1/4 cup almond butter
- ✓ 3 packets or 1 1/2 tsp. powdered stevia

**_Preparation:_**

1. Preheat the oven to 375°F (190°C).
2. Grease a 12-cup muffin tray or use paper liners.
3. In a large bowl, whisk together the buckwheat flour, ground flaxseed, baking powder, cinnamon, and salt.
4. In a separate bowl, whisk together the eggs, unsweetened almond milk, almond butter, and powdered stevia.
5. Stir the wet and dry ingredients together until thoroughly blended.
6. Evenly divide the batter among the muffin cups that have been prepared.
7. Bake for 20–25 minutes, or until a toothpick inserted into the middle of a muffin comes out clean.

8. Allow the muffins to cool in the pan for 5 minutes before transferring them to a wire rack to cool fully.

***Nutritional Value (per muffin):*** Calories: 120, Fat: 6g, Carbohydrates: 12g, Fiber: 2g, Protein: 4g, Sodium: 120mg.

***Prep Time:*** 30 minutes

**N**ote: These Buckwheat Breakfast Muffins are a delicious and nutritious breakfast option that is suitable for the Candida diet. They are gluten-free, sugar-free, and packed with protein, fiber, and healthy fats.

# Crunchy, Chunky Cinnamon Pecan Granola

***Ingredients:***

- ✓ 2 cups rolled oats
- ✓ 1 cup chopped pecans
- ✓ 1/4 cup unsweetened shredded coconut
- ✓ 1/4 cup ground flaxseed
- ✓ 1/4 cup coconut oil, melted
- ✓ 1/4 cup powdered stevia
- ✓ 1 tsp. ground cinnamon
- ✓ 1/4 tsp. salt
- ✓ 1/4 cup sugar-free maple syrup

***Preparation:***

1. Preheat the oven to 300°F (150°C).
2. Use parchment paper to line a baking tray.

3. In a large bowl, combine the rolled oats, chopped pecans, unsweetened shredded coconut, ground flaxseed, ground cinnamon, and salt. Mix well.

4. In a separate bowl, whisk together the melted coconut oil, powdered stevia, and sugar-free maple syrup.

5. Pour the liquid mixture over the dry ingredients and whisk until thoroughly incorporated.

6. Toss the ingredients onto the baking sheet and spread them out evenly.

7. Bake for 30–35 minutes, stirring every 10 minutes, until the granola turns golden and crunchy.

8. Allow the granola to set completely on the baking tray.

9. Once chilled, keep the granola in an airtight container.

***Nutritional Value (per serving, 1/2 cup):*** Calories: 220,Fat: 18g, Carbohydrates: 12g, Fiber: 4g, Protein: 5g, Sodium: 60mg.

***Prep Time:*** 45 minutes

**N**ote: This crunchy, chunky cinnamon pecan granola is a delicious and nutritious breakfast option that is suitable for the Candida diet. It is gluten-free, sugar-free, and packed with healthy fats, fiber, and essential nutrients.

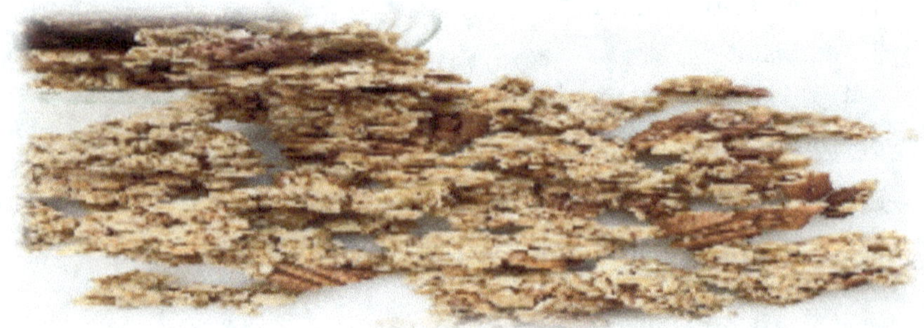

# Healthy Almond Flour Pumpkin Muffins

## *Ingredients:*

- ✓ 2 cups of almond flour
- ✓ 1 tsp. baking soda
- ✓ 1 tbsp. pumpkin pie spice
- ✓ 1/2 tsp. ground cinnamon
- ✓ 1/4 tsp. salt
- ✓ 2/3 cup canned pumpkin
- ✓ 2 large eggs
- ✓ 1/4 cup honey or maple syrup
- ✓ 1 tbsp. coconut oil, melted
- ✓ 1 tsp. vanilla extract

## *Preparation:*

1. Preheat the oven to 350°F (175°C).
2. Use paper liners to line a muffin pan.
3. In a large bowl, whisk together the almond flour, baking soda, pumpkin pie spice, cinnamon, and salt.
4. In a separate bowl, whisk together the canned pumpkin, eggs, honey or maple syrup, coconut oil, and vanilla extract.
5. Stir the wet and dry ingredients together until thoroughly blended.
6. Evenly divide the batter among the muffin cups that have been prepared.

7. Bake for 20–25 minutes, or until a toothpick inserted into the middle of a muffin comes out clean.

8. Allow the muffins to cool in the pan for 5 minutes before transferring them to a wire rack to cool fully.

***Nutritional Value (per muffin):*** Calories: 180, Fat: 12g, Carbohydrates: 15g, Fiber: 3g, Protein: 6g, Sugar: 8g, Sodium: 180mg.

***Prep Time:*** 30 minutes

**N**ote: These healthy almond-flour pumpkin muffins are a delicious and nutritious breakfast option that is suitable for the Candida diet. They are gluten-free, sugar-free, and packed with healthy fats, fiber, and essential nutrients.

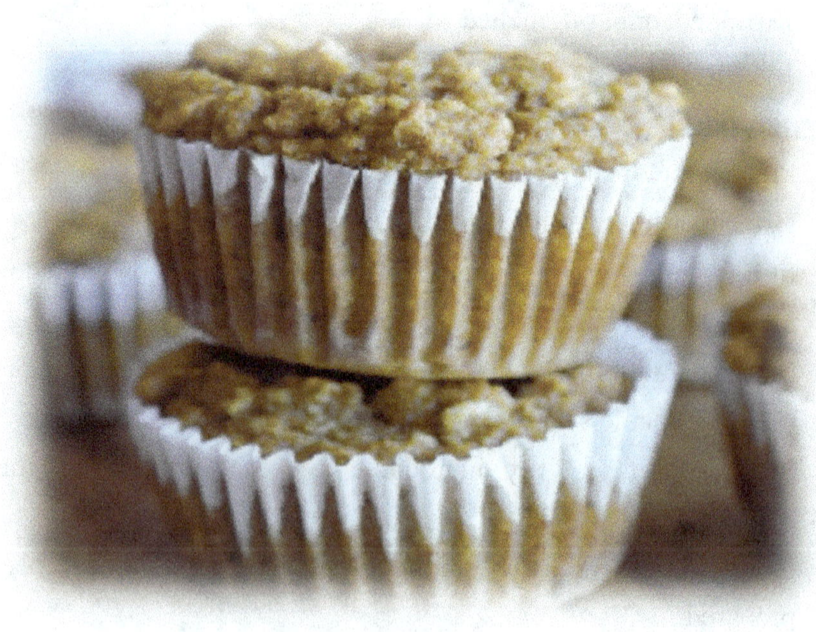

# CHAPTER 3
## CANDIDA-FRIENDLY LUNCH RECIPES FOR WELLNESS

## Chicken and Vegetable Soup

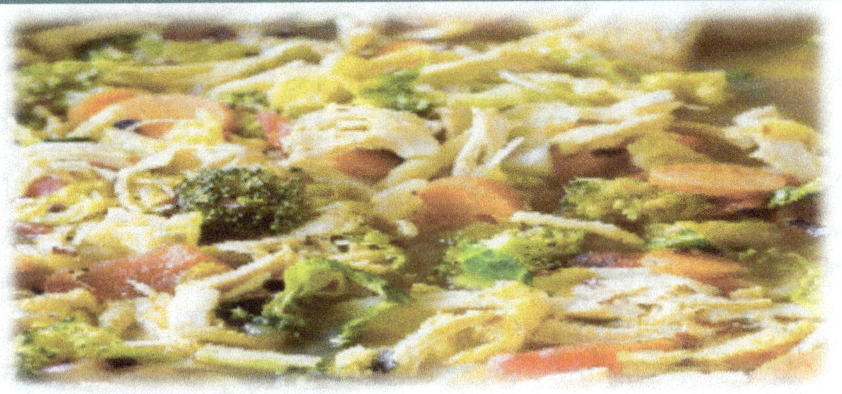

### *Ingredients:*

- ✓ 2 tbsp. ghee
- ✓ 1 medium onion, diced
- ✓ 4 garlic cloves, minced
- ✓ 8 oz. mushrooms, sliced
- ✓ 1 cup carrots, cut into bite-size pieces
- ✓ 4 cups of chicken broth
- ✓ 1 cup cooked chicken, shredded
- ✓ 1 cup kale, chopped
- ✓ 1 tsp. dried thyme

✓  1 tsp. dried rosemary

✓  Salt and pepper to taste

***Preparation:***

1.  In a large saucepan, heat the ghee over average heat.
2.  Add the diced onion and garlic to the saucepan.
3.  Sauté the onion for 5 minutes, or until it starts to become translucent.
4.  Add the sliced mushrooms and carrots to the saucepan.
5.  Cook the veggies for 5 minutes, or until tender.
6.  Add the chicken broth, cooked chicken, chopped kale, dried thyme, and dried rosemary to the pot. Stir to combine.
7.  Bring the soup to a boil, then reduce the heat and simmer for 20–25 minutes, or until the vegetables are tender and the flavors have melded.
8.  Season with salt and pepper, to taste.
9.  Serve the soup hot and enjoy!

Nutritional Value (per serving): Calories: 180, Fat: 8g, Carbohydrates: 10g, Fiber: 2g, Protein: 18g, Sugar: 4g, Sodium: 480mg.

***Prep Time:*** 45 minutes

**N**ote: This chicken and vegetable soup is a delicious and nutritious lunch option that is suitable for the Candida diet. It is gluten-free, sugar-free, and packed with protein, fiber, and essential nutrients.

# Zucchini Noodles With Pesto

## Ingredients:

- ✓ 4 medium zucchinis, spiralized
- ✓ 1/2 cup of fresh basil leaves
- ✓ 1/4 cup pine nuts
- ✓ 2 garlic cloves, minced
- ✓ 1/4 cup olive oil
- ✓ 1/4 cup nutritional yeast
- ✓ Salt and pepper to taste

## Preparation:

1. In a food processor, combine the fresh basil leaves, pine nuts, minced garlic, olive oil, and nutritional yeast. Pulse until the mixture is smooth and creamy.
2. Add salt and pepper to the pesto as desired.
3. In a large skillet, heat a little bit of olive oil over medium heat.
4. Add the spiralized zucchini noodles to the skillet and sauté for 2-3 minutes, or until the noodles are tender.
5. Add the pesto to the skillet and toss to coat the zucchini noodles evenly.
6. Cook for an additional 1-2 minutes, or until the pesto is heated through.
7. Serve the zucchini noodles hot and enjoy!

<u>**_Nutritional Value (per serving):_**</u> Calories: 180, Fat: 16g, Carbohydrates: 8g, Fiber: 3g, Protein: 5g; Sugar: 4g, Sodium: 80mg.

<u>**_Prep Time:_**</u> 20 minutes

**N**ote: These Zucchini Noodles with Pesto are a delicious and nutritious lunch option that is suitable for the Candida diet. They are gluten-free, sugar-free, and packed with healthy fats, fiber, and essential nutrients

# Grilled Chicken Salad With Avocado

<u>**_Ingredients:_**</u>

- ✓ 1 skinless chicken breast
- ✓ 1/2 tsp. paprika
- ✓ 1/2 tsp. garlic powder
- ✓ 1/2 teaspoon chili powder
- ✓ 1/2 tsp. cumin
- ✓ 1 tbsp. olive oil
- ✓ 2 cups of spinach
- ✓ 2 medium tomatoes
- ✓ 1/2 cucumber
- ✓ 1 avocado
- ✓ 2 shallots
- ✓ 1 garlic clove, minced
- ✓ Juice of 1/2 lemon

✓ 2 tbsp. olive oil

✓ Sea salt

### *Preparation:*

1. In a small bowl, mix the paprika, garlic powder, chili powder, and cumin.
2. Apply the spice mixture to the chicken breast.
3. In a skillet, heat the olive oil over medium-high heat.
4. Add the chicken breast and cook for 6-7 minutes on each side, or until the chicken is no longer pink in the center.
5. Remove it from the skillet and let it rest for 5 minutes. Slice the chicken.
6. In a large bowl, combine the spinach, tomatoes, cucumber, avocado, and shallots.
7. In a small bowl, whisk together the minced garlic, lemon juice, and olive oil. Season with sea salt.
8. Pour the dressing over the salad and toss to combine.
9. Top the salad with the sliced grilled chicken.

***Nutritional Value (per serving):*** Calories: 380, Fat: 24g, Carbohydrates: 18g, Fiber: 8g, Protein: 28g, Sugar: 6g, Sodium: 120mg.

***Prep Time:*** 25 minutes

**N**ote: This Grilled chicken Salad with Avocado is a delicious and nutritious lunch option that is suitable for the Candida diet. It is gluten-free, sugar-free, and packed with healthy fats, fiber, and essential nutrients.

# Turkey and Vegetable Stir-Fry

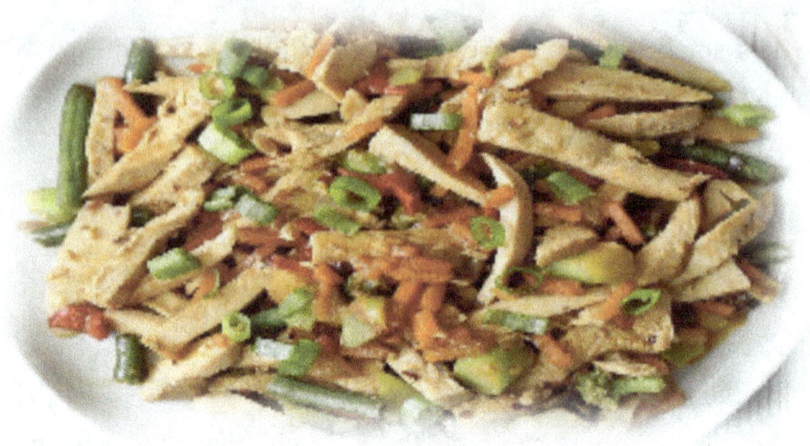

### *Ingredients:*

- ✓ 1 lb. ground turkey
- ✓ 1/2 cup minced onion
- ✓ 1 clove of garlic, thinly sliced
- ✓ 1 tsp. allspice
- ✓ 2 tsp. cumin
- ✓ 1 tsp. salt
- ✓ Pinch of pepper
- ✓ 2 cups roughly chopped chard leaves
- ✓ 2 cups thinly sliced green cabbage
- ✓ 2 Tbsp. minced fresh mint
- ✓ 1 orange bell pepper, sliced into strips
- ✓ Zest of 1 lemon

✓ 1 Tbsp. lemon juice

✓ Olive or coconut oil for cooking

***Preparation:***

1. In a large skillet over medium heat, add a little bit of oil (olive or coconut oil) and sauté the minced onion and sliced garlic until the garlic is fragrant.

2. Add the ground turkey to the skillet and cook until browned, about 7-8 minutes.

3. Add the allspice, cumin, salt, and pepper to the skillet and stir to combine.

4. Add the roughly chopped chard leaves, thinly sliced green cabbage, and orange bell pepper strips to the skillet.

5. Sauté until the chard and cabbage have wilted and the pepper strips have softened, about 3 minutes.

6. Add the zest of 1 lemon and 1 tablespoon of lemon juice to the skillet and stir to combine.

7. Remove from heat and stir in the minced fresh mint.

***Nutritional Value (per serving):*** Calories: 250, Fat: 12g, Carbohydrates: 10g, Fiber: 3g, Protein: 25g, Sugar: 3g, Sodium: 500mg.

***Prep Time:*** 25 minutes

Note: This Turkey and Vegetable Stir-Fry is a delicious and nutritious lunch option that is suitable for the Candida diet. It is gluten-free, sugar-free, and packed with healthy fats, fiber, and essential nutrients.

# Roasted Cauliflower and Broccoli Salad

### *Ingredients:*

- ✓ 1 head of cauliflower, cut into florets
- ✓ 2 heads of broccoli, cut into florets
- ✓ 2-3 tablespoons of olive oil
- ✓ 1 teaspoon garlic powder
- ✓ 1 teaspoon of onion powder
- ✓ Salt and pepper to taste
- ✓ 1/4 cup chopped fresh parsley
- ✓ 2 tablespoons of lemon juice
- ✓ 1/4 cup toasted pumpkin seeds (optional)

### *Preparation:*

1. Preheat the oven to 425°F (220°C).
2. In a large bowl, toss the cauliflower and broccoli florets with olive oil, garlic powder, onion powder, salt, and pepper until evenly coated.
3. Place the florets in a single layer on a baking pan.
4. Roast for 25–30 minutes, or until the vegetables are tender and golden brown, stirring once halfway through.
5. Let the vegetables cool to room temperature after removing them from the oven.
6. In a large serving bowl, combine the roasted cauliflower and broccoli.

7. Add the chopped fresh parsley, lemon juice, and toasted pumpkin seeds (if using). Toss gently to combine.

***Nutritional Value (per serving):*** Calories: 180, Fat: 10g, Carbohydrates: 20, Fiber: 8g, Protein: 8g, Sugar: 6g, Sodium: 300mg.

***Prep Time:*** 35 minutes

**N**ote: This roasted cauliflower and broccoli salad is a delicious and nutritious lunch option that is suitable for the Candida diet. It is gluten-free, sugar-free, and packed with healthy fats, fiber, and essential nutrients.

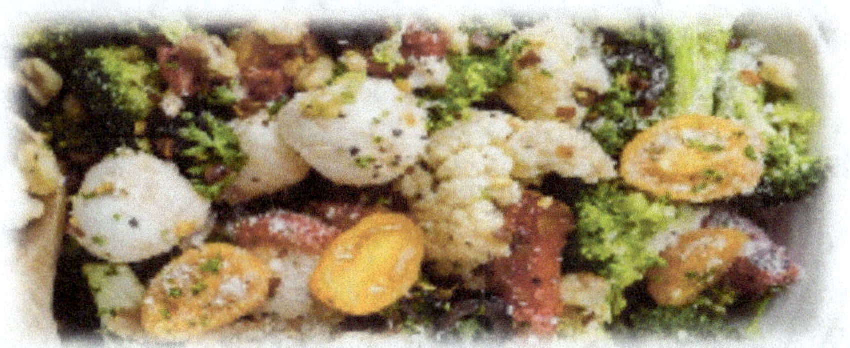

# Spicy Shrimp and Vegetable Stir-Fry

***Ingredients:***

- ✓ 1 lb. shrimp, peeled and deveined
- ✓ 1 red bell pepper, sliced
- ✓ 1 yellow bell pepper, sliced
- ✓ 1 zucchini, sliced

✓  1 yellow squash, sliced

✓  1/2 onion, sliced

✓  2 garlic cloves, minced

✓  1 teaspoon ginger, minced

✓  1/4 cup coconut aminos

✓  1 tbsp apple cider vinegar

✓  1 tsp. honey

✓  1 tsp. red pepper flakes

✓  2 tbsp. olive oil

✓  Salt and pepper to taste

### *Preparation:*

1. In a small bowl, whisk together the coconut aminos, apple cider vinegar, honey, and red pepper flakes. Set aside.
2. Heat the olive oil in a big pan or wok until it is very hot.
3. In a pan, combine the minced garlic, ginger, and sliced onion.
4. Cook for 1–2 minutes, or until aromatic.
5. Add the sliced bell peppers, zucchini, and yellow squash to the pan.
6. Sauté for 3–4 minutes, or until the veggies are soft and crispy.
7. Add the shrimp to the skillet and sauté for 2-3 minutes, or until the shrimp are pink and cooked through.
8. Pour the coconut aminos mixture over the stir-fry and toss to coat the vegetables and shrimp evenly.
9. Add salt and pepper to taste.
10. Serve the spicy shrimp and vegetable stir-fry hot and enjoy!

<u>***Nutritional Value (per serving):***</u> Calories: 250, Fat: 10, Carbohydrates: 15g, Fiber: 4g, Protein: 25g, Sugar: 8, Sodium: 600mg.

<u>***Prep Time:***</u> 30 minutes

**N**ote: This spicy shrimp and vegetable stir-fry is a delicious and nutritious lunch option that is suitable for the Candida diet. It is gluten-free, sugar-free, and packed with protein, fiber, and essential nutrients.

# Creamy Broccoli Soup

## <u>*Ingredients:*</u>

✓ 1 lb. broccoli, stems diced, florets chopped

✓ 2 cups original or unsweetened non-dairy milk (e.g., cashew milk)

✓ 3/4 cup full-fat canned coconut milk

✓ 1/4 cup of nutritional yeast flakes

✓ 1 tsp. white wine vinegar or lemon juice

✓ 1/2 teaspoon salt, to taste

✓ Black pepper, to taste

✓ 1 cup of broccoli florets

✓ 1 tbsp. olive oil

✓ Salt, to taste

## <u>*Preparation:*</u>

1. In a medium saucepan, heat the olive oil over average heat.

2. Add the diced broccoli, carrots, and garlic.

3. Cook the veggies for 5 minutes, or until they're soft.

4. Add the vegetable broth, non-dairy milk, coconut milk, and nutritional yeast.

5. Bring to a simmer and cook for 15 minutes, or until the broccoli is very tender.

6. Using an immersion blender, blend the soup until smooth.

7. Add salt and pepper to taste.

8. In a small skillet, heat the olive oil over medium heat.

9. Add the broccoli florets and sauté until they are bright green and lightly browned. Season with salt.

***Nutritional Value (per serving):*** Calories: 180, Fat: 10g, Carbohydrates: 15g, Fiber: 5g, Protein: 8g, Sugar: 6g, Sodium: 600mg.

***Prep Time:*** 30 minutes

**N**ote: This creamy broccoli soup is a delicious and nutritious lunch option that is suitable for the Candida diet. It is gluten-free, sugar-free, and packed with healthy fats, fiber, and essential nutrients.

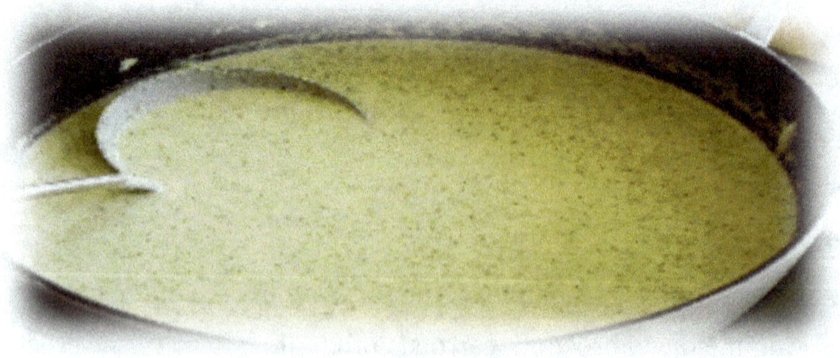

# Grilled Salmon With Asparagus

### Ingredients:

- ✓ 2 (3 oz.) fillets of wild salmon
- ✓ 1 garlic clove, grated
- ✓ 1 tbsp. chopped parsley
- ✓ 2 tbsp extra-virgin olive oil
- ✓ 2 tbsp. fresh lemon juice
- ✓ Salt and pepper to taste
- ✓ 1 lb. asparagus, trimmed
- ✓ 1 tbsp. olive oil

### Preparation:

1. In a glass bowl, whisk together all of the ingredients for the marinade.
2. Sprinkle the salmon with a little bit of sea salt and pepper.
3. Marinade the fish and place it in the fridge for 10 minutes while you heat the grill.
4. Heat a lightly oiled grill and cook the salmon for 3–4 minutes on each side, or until the fish is cooked through.
5. In a separate pan, heat the olive oil over medium-high heat. Add the asparagus and sauté for 5-7 minutes, or until the asparagus is tender-crisp.
6. Add salt and pepper to the asparagus as desired.
7. Serve the grilled salmon with the sautéed asparagus, and enjoy!

<u>**Nutritional Value (per serving):**</u> Calories: 300, Fat: 20g, Carbohydrates: 6g, Fiber: 3g, Protein: 25g, Sugar: 3g, Sodium: 200mg.

<u>**Prep Time:**</u> 20 minutes

**N**ote: This grilled salmon with asparagus is a delicious and nutritious lunch option that is suitable for the Candida diet. It is gluten-free, sugar-free, and packed with healthy fats, fiber, and essential nutrients.

# Turkey and Vegetable Lettuce Wraps

<u>**Ingredients:**</u>

- ✓ 1 lb. ground turkey
- ✓ 1 tsp. garlic powder
- ✓ 1 tsp. cumin
- ✓ 1 tsp. salt
- ✓ 1 tsp. chili powder
- ✓ 1 tsp. paprika
- ✓ 1/2 tsp. oregano
- ✓ 1/2 small onion, minced
- ✓ 2 tbsp. minced bell pepper
- ✓ 3/4 cup water
- ✓ 4 oz. cans of tomato sauce
- ✓ 8 large lettuce leaves from Iceberg lettuce

✓ 1/2 cup shredded reduced-fat cheddar (optional; omit for Whole30)

## Preparation:

1. Brown the turkey in a large skillet, breaking it into smaller pieces as it cooks.

2. When the mixture is no longer pink, add the dry seasoning and combine thoroughly.

3. Add the tomato sauce, onion, pepper, and water.

4. Sauté on low for around 20 minutes.

5. Wash and dry the lettuce leaves. Ensure they are crisp and pliable.

**Nutritional Value (per serving):** Calories: 180, Fat: 8g, Carbohydrates: 6g, Fiber: 2g, Protein: 20g, Sugar: 3g, Sodium: 400mg.

**Prep Time:** 30 minutes

Note: This Turkey and Vegetable Lettuce Wraps recipe is a delicious and nutritious lunch option that is suitable for the Candida diet. It is gluten-free, sugar-free, and packed with protein, fiber, and essential nutrients.

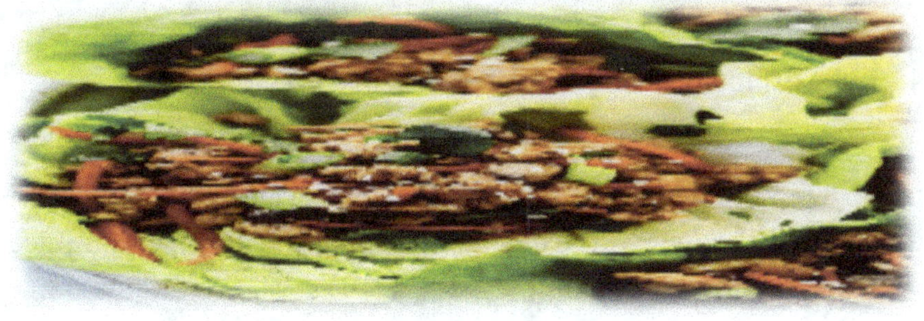

# Quinoa and Vegetable Salad

**_Ingredients:_**

- ✓ 1/2 cup uncooked quinoa
- ✓ 2 cups of spinach
- ✓ 2 medium tomatoes
- ✓ 1/2 cucumber
- ✓ 1 avocado
- ✓ 2 shallots
- ✓ 1 garlic clove, minced
- ✓ Juice of 1/2 lemon
- ✓ 2 Tbsp. olive oil
- ✓ Sea salt

**_Preparation:_**

1. Rinse the quinoa in cold water.
2. In an averageIn a average a saucepan, mix the quinoa and 1 cup of water.
3. Bring to a boil, then reduce the heat to low, cover, and simmer for 15 minutes, or until the quinoa is tender and the water is absorbed.
4. Take off the heat and leave to cool.
5. In a large bowl, combine the cooked quinoa, spinach, diced tomatoes, sliced cucumber, diced avocado, and minced shallots.
6. In a small bowl, whisk together the minced garlic, lemon juice, and olive oil. Season with sea salt.

7. Pour the dressing over the quinoa and vegetable mixture and toss gently to combine.

***Nutritional Value (per serving):*** Calories: 320, Fat: 18g, Carbohydrates: 32g, Fiber: 8g, Protein: 9g, Sugar: 4g, Sodium: 150mg.

***Prep Time:*** 25 minutes

**N**ote: This Quinoa and Vegetable Salad is a delicious and nutritious lunch option that is suitable for the Candida diet. It is gluten-free, sugar-free, and packed with healthy fats, fiber, and essential nutrients.

# Baked Chicken With Roasted Vegetables

## *Ingredients:*

- ✓ 2 boneless, skinless chicken breasts
- ✓ 1/2 lb. asparagus, trimmed
- ✓ 1/2 lb. cherry tomatoes
- ✓ 1/2 red onion, sliced
- ✓ 2 garlic cloves, minced
- ✓ 2 tbsp. olive oil
- ✓ 1 tsp. dried oregano
- ✓ 1 tsp. dried basil
- ✓ Salt and pepper to taste

## *Preparation:*

- ✓ Preheat the oven to 400°F (200°C).

✓ In a large bowl, toss the asparagus, cherry tomatoes, red onion, and minced garlic with olive oil, dried oregano, dried basil, salt, and pepper until evenly coated.

✓ Place the vegetables on a baking sheet in a single layer.

✓ Place the chicken breasts on the vegetables.

✓ Add salt and pepper to the chicken breasts as desired.

✓ Bake for 25–30 minutes, or until the chicken is cooked through and the vegetables are tender and golden brown.

***Nutritional Value (per serving):*** Calories: 300, Fat: 14g, Carbohydrates: 10g, Fiber: 3g, Protein: 35g, Sugar: 5g, Sodium: 200mg.

***Prep Time:*** 35 minutes

**N**ote: This Baked Chicken with Roasted Vegetables recipe is a delicious and nutritious lunch option that is suitable for the Candida diet. It is gluten-free, sugar-free, and packed with protein, fiber, and essential nutrients.

# *Cucumber and Avocado Soup*

***Ingredients:***

✓ 2 medium cucumbers, peeled and chopped

✓ 1 avocado, peeled and pitted

✓ 1 garlic clove, minced

✓ 1/4 cup fresh cilantro, chopped

✓ 1/4 cup fresh parsley, chopped

✓ 1/4 cup fresh mint, chopped

✓ 1/4 cup of lemon juice

✓ 1/4 cup extra-virgin olive oil

✓ 1/2 tsp. sea salt

✓ 1/4 tsp. black pepper

✓ 1/2 cup of water

***Preparation:***

1. In a blender or food processor, combine the chopped cucumbers, avocado, minced garlic, chopped cilantro, chopped parsley, chopped mint, lemon juice, olive oil, sea salt, black pepper, and water.

2. Blend until smooth and creamy.

3. Taste and adjust the seasoning as needed.

4. Before serving, cool the soup for at least 30 minutes in the refrigerator.

***Nutritional Value (per serving):*** Calories: 250, Fat: 22, Carbohydrates: 12g, Fiber: 7g, Protein: 4g, Sugar: 3g, Sodium: 300mg.

***Prep Time:*** 10 minutes

**N**ote: This cucumber and avocado soup is a delicious and nutritious lunch option that is suitable for the Candida diet. It is gluten-free, sugar-free, and packed with healthy fats, fiber, and essential nutrients.

# *Tuna Salad With Avocado*

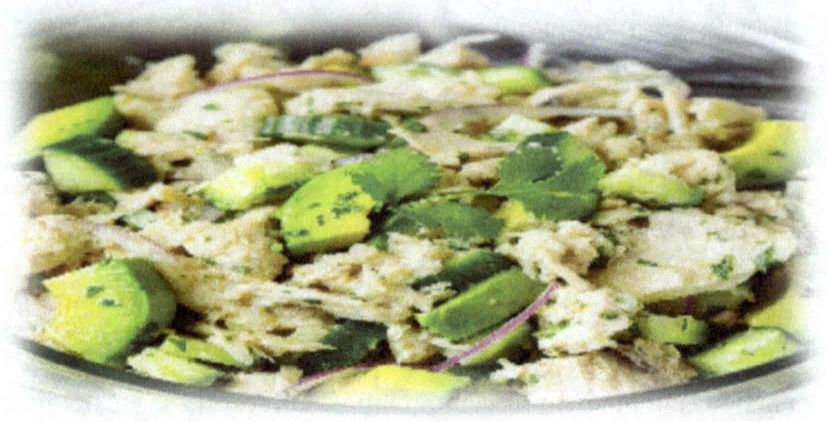

## *Ingredients:*

- ✓  1 (5 oz.) can of wild albacore tuna
- ✓  1 small or medium avocado
- ✓  1 carrot, chopped
- ✓  1 celery stalk, chopped
- ✓  2 tbsp. lemon juice
- ✓  Salt and pepper to taste

## *Preparation:*

1. In a medium bowl, combine the drained tuna, mashed avocado, chopped carrot, chopped celery, lemon juice, salt, and pepper.
2. Mix well until all components are equally combined.
3. Serve the tuna salad on a bed of lettuce or with gluten-free crackers.

<u>**Nutritional Value (per serving):**</u> Calories: 250, Fat: 15g, Carbohydrates: 12g, Fiber: 7g, Protein: 20g, Sugar: 3g, Sodium: 300mg.

<u>**Prep Time:**</u> 10 minute

<u>**Note:**</u> This tuna salad with avocado recipe is a delicious and nutritious lunch option that is suitable for the Candida diet. It is gluten-free, sugar-free, and packed with healthy fats, fiber, and essential nutrients.

# Grilled Shrimp and Vegetable Skewers

<u>**Ingredients:**</u>

- ✓  1 lb. large shrimp, peeled and deveined
- ✓  1 red bell pepper, sliced
- ✓  1 yellow bell pepper, sliced
- ✓  1 zucchini, sliced
- ✓  1 yellow squash, sliced
- ✓  1/2 onion, sliced
- ✓  2 garlic cloves, minced
- ✓  2 tbsp. olive oil
- ✓  Salt and pepper to taste

<u>**Preparation:**</u>

1. Preheat the grill to medium-high heat.

2. Thread the shrimp, sliced bell peppers, sliced zucchini, sliced yellow squash, and sliced onion onto skewers.

3. In a small bowl, combine the garlic, olive oil, salt, and pepper.

4. Brush the skewers with the garlic and olive oil mixture.

5. Grill the skewers for 2-3 minutes on each side, or until the shrimp are pink and opaque and the vegetables are tender and golden brown.

**_Nutritional Value (per serving):_** Calories: 250, Fat: 12g, Carbohydrates: 10g, Fiber: 3g, Protein: 25, Sugar: 5g, Sodium: 200mg.

**_Prep Time:_** 30 minutes

**N**ote: This Grilled Shrimp and Vegetable Skewers recipe is a delicious and nutritious lunch option that is suitable for the Candida diet. It is gluten-free, sugar-free, and packed with protein, fiber, and essential nutrients.

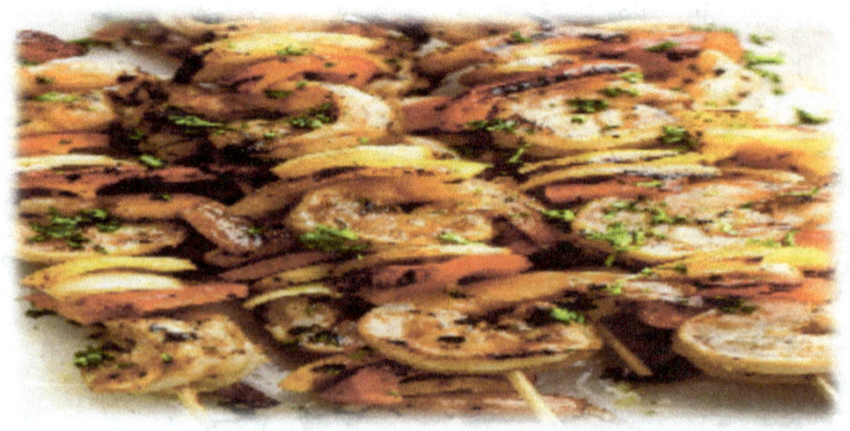

# CHAPTER 4

## CANDIDA-FRIENDLY RECIPES FOR A NOURISHING DINNERS

### Curried Cauliflower Soup

**Ingredients:**

- ✓ 1 lb. cauliflower, cut into bite-size pieces (about 1 small cauliflower)
- ✓ 4 tablespoons of oil, such as melted coconut oil or olive oil, separated
- ✓ Salt and pepper
- ✓ 1/2 medium onion, diced
- ✓ 1 clove of garlic, sliced
- ✓ 1/2 tsp. powdered cumin
- ✓ 1/2 tsp. powdered ginger
- ✓ 1/2 tsp. powdered turmeric
- ✓ 1/4 tsp. red pepper flakes
- ✓ 1 can (14 oz.) of coconut milk
- ✓ 2 cups vegetable or chicken broth
- ✓ Fresh cilantro, for garnish
- ✓ Lime wedges, for serving

**Preparation:**

1. Preheat your oven to 425°F.

2. Toss the cauliflower with 2 tablespoons of the oil and season with salt and pepper.
3. Spread the cauliflower on a baking sheet and roast for 20–25 minutes, or until it's golden brown.
4. In a large pot, heat the remaining 2 tablespoons of oil over medium heat.
5. Cook the onion for approximately 5 minutes, or until tender and transparent.
6. Add the garlic, cumin, ginger, turmeric, and red pepper flakes, and cook for 1 minute.
7. Add the roasted cauliflower, coconut milk, and broth to the pot.
8. After bringing the soup to a boil, lower the heat and simmer it for 20 minutes.
9. Use an immersion blender to smooth up the soup.
10. If you do not have an immersion blender, you may use a conventional blender to make the soup in batches.
11. Spice the soup to taste with salt and pepper.
12. If the soup is too thick, add additional liquid to thin it up.
13. Serve the soup with a garnish of fresh cilantro and a lime wedge on the side.

***Nutritional Value (per serving):*** Calories: 250, Fat: 15g, Carbohydrates: 12g, Fiber: 7, Protein: 4g, Sugar: 3g, Sodium: 300mg.

***Prep Time:*** 10 minutes

***Total Cooking Time:*** 45 minutes

Note: This curried cauliflower soup recipe is a delicious and nutritious dinner option that is suitable for the Candida diet. It is gluten-free, sugar-free, and packed with healthy fats, fiber, and essential nutrients.

## Toasted Coconut and Lime Salmon

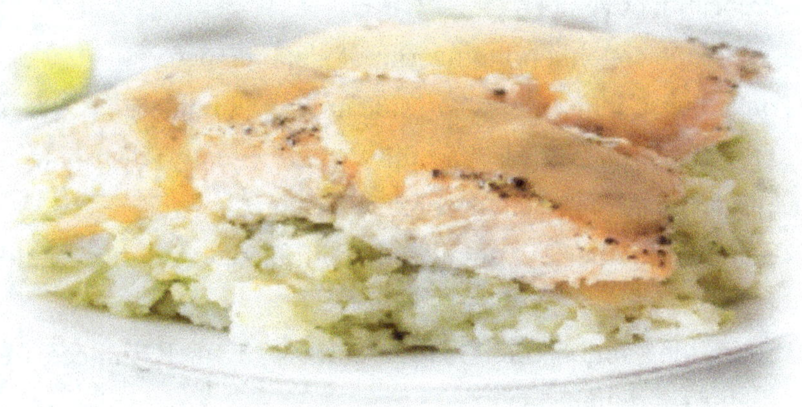

### Ingredients:

- ✓ 2 (4 oz.) wild-caught salmon fillets
- ✓ 2 Tbsp. fresh lime juice
- ✓ 2 Tbsp. coconut aminos
- ✓ 1/4 tsp. chili powder
- ✓ 1/4 tsp. salt
- ✓ 1 Tbsp. coconut oil
- ✓ 2 Tbsp. unsweetened shredded coconut

✓ Fresh cilantro, finely minced

✓ Lime slices, for serving

***Preparation:***

1. In a shallow dish, whisk together the lime juice, coconut aminos, chili powder, and salt.
2. Add the salmon fillets to the marinade, skin side up, and let them marinate for 30 minutes.
3. Preheat the oven to 425°F (218°C).
4. Apply the coconut oil to the rim of a baking pan.
5. Bake the salmon fillets, skin side up, for 5 minutes.
6. Turn the fillets over carefully, then equally distribute the unsweetened shredded coconut over top.
7. Bake for another 2-3 minutes, or until the coconut turns golden brown.
8. Serve the salmon fillets with a garnish of finely minced fresh cilantro and lime slices.

Nutritional Value (per serving): Calories: 25, Fat: 15g, Carbohydrates: 5g, Fiber: 2g, Protein: 25g, Sugar: 1g, Sodium: 400mg.

***Prep Time:*** 35 minutes

**N**ote: This toasted coconut and lime salmon recipe is a delicious and nutritious dinner option that is suitable for the Candida diet. It is gluten-free, sugar-free, and packed with healthy fats, fiber, and essential nutrients.

# Arugula and Tomato Salad With Tomato Vinaigrette

## Ingredients:

- ✓ 4 cups of arugula
- ✓ 1 cucumber, sliced into rounds
- ✓ 1 cup cherry tomatoes, halved
- ✓ 1 avocado, peeled, seeded, and sliced
- ✓ 3 to 4 fresh cherry tomatoes, chopped
- ✓ 1/2 cup oil, such as olive or avocado
- ✓ 1/4 cup apple cider vinegar
- ✓ 2 Tbsp. coconut aminos
- ✓ 1 clove of garlic, finely minced
- ✓ 1 tsp. dried oregano
- ✓ Salt and pepper to taste

## Preparation:

1. To prepare the vinaigrette, combine the diced cherry tomatoes, oil, apple cider vinegar, coconut aminos, minced garlic, and dried oregano in a blender.

2. Process till smooth, and add salt and pepper to taste.

3. To make the salad, add the arugula, sliced cucumber rounds, and cherry tomato halves into a large salad bowl and toss to combine.

4. Drizzle the salad with the tomato vinaigrette, and garnish with the avocado slices. Serve immediately.

<u>**Nutritional Value (per serving):**</u> Calories: 200, Fat: 15g, Carbohydrates: 10g, Fiber: 5g, Protein: 4g, Sugar: 3g, Sodium: 200mg.

<u>**Prep Time:**</u> 10 minutes

**N**ote: This Arugula and Tomato Salad with Tomato Vinaigrette recipe is a delicious and nutritious dinner option that is suitable for the Candida diet. It is gluten-free, sugar-free, and packed with healthy fats, fiber, and essential nutrients.

# Almond-Crusted Chicken Fingers

<u>**Ingredients:**</u>

- ✓ 1 ½ pounds boneless and skinless chicken breasts or tenders, cut into 1 ½-inch strips
- ✓ 1 cup of almond meal
- ✓ ½ teaspoon cayenne pepper (optional)
- ✓ ¼ cup desiccated coconut
- ✓ 1 teaspoon garlic powder
- ✓ 2 tablespoons of flaxseed meal
- ✓ 4 large egg whites
- ✓ 2 tablespoons of coconut oil
- ✓ Salt and pepper to taste

<u>**Preparation:**</u>

1. Preheat the oven to 425°F (218°C).

2. In a medium bowl, mix together the almond meal, cayenne pepper (if using), desiccated coconut, garlic powder, and flaxseed meal.

3. In a separate bowl, whisk the egg whites until they are frothy.

4. Dip the chicken pieces in the egg whites and coat them with the dry mixture, shaking off any excess.

5. Place the coated chicken pieces on a prepared baking sheet.

6. Bake for about 25 minutes, turning once, until the chicken fingers are golden brown and crisp.

7. In an average mixing bowl, combine yogurt, garlic powder, chives, lime zest, and juice. Season to taste.

8. Serve the chicken fingers with the dip and a salad or some sliced avocado.

***Nutritional Value (per serving):*** Calories: 250, Fat: 15g, Carbohydrates: 5g, Fiber: 2g, Protein: 25g, Sugar: 1g, Sodium: 400mg.

***Prep Time:*** 35 minutes

**N**ote: This almond-crusted chicken finger recipe is a delicious and nutritious dinner option that is suitable for the Candida diet. It is gluten-free, sugar-free, and packed with healthy fats, fiber, and essential nutrients.

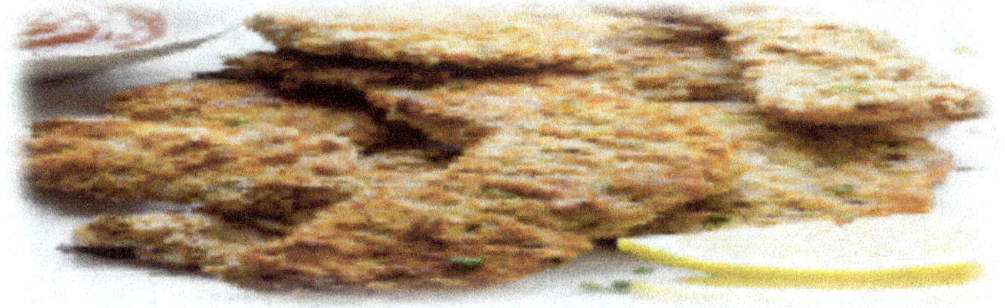

# Rutabaga and Rosemary Bread

## Ingredients:

- ✓ 1 cup rutabaga puree
- ✓ 1/2 Tbsp. oil, olive, or coconut (melted)
- ✓ 4 eggs
- ✓ 1 tsp. apple cider vinegar
- ✓ 3 cups of almond flour
- ✓ 1/2 cup coconut flour, sifted
- ✓ 1 tsp. baking soda
- ✓ 1 tsp. salt
- ✓ Pepper to taste
- ✓ 1 Tbsp. fresh rosemary, finely minced

## Preparation:

1. Preheat the oven to 350°F (175°C).
2. Peel and chop a big rutabaga (approximately 1 1/2 pounds) into 1-inch cubes.
3. Place in a medium saucepan with a pinch of salt, then add enough water just to cover the rutabaga. Bring to a boil, then reduce the heat and simmer for 20–25 minutes, or until the rutabaga is tender.
4. Drain the rutabaga and puree it in a food processor or blender until smooth.

5. In a large bowl, combine the rutabaga puree, oil, eggs, and apple cider vinegar. Mix well.

6. In a separate bowl, whisk together the almond flour, coconut flour, baking soda, salt, pepper, and minced rosemary.

7. Add the dry ingredients to the wet ingredients and mix until well combined.

8. Pour the batter into a greased loaf pan, and level the surface with a spatula.

9. Bake the bread for 45–50 minutes, or until a toothpick put in the middle comes out clean.

10. Let the bread cool in the pan for 10 minutes, then remove it from the pan and let it cool completely on a wire rack before slicing.

**_Nutritional Value (per serving):_** Calories: 200, Fat: 15g, Carbohydrates: 10g, Fiber: 5g, Protein: 8g, Sugar: 2g, Sodium: 300mg.

**_Prep Time:_** 1 hour

**N**ote: This Rutabaga and Rosemary Bread recipe is a delicious and nutritious dinner option that is suitable for the Candida diet. It is gluten-free, sugar-free, and packed with healthy fats, fiber, and essential nutrients.

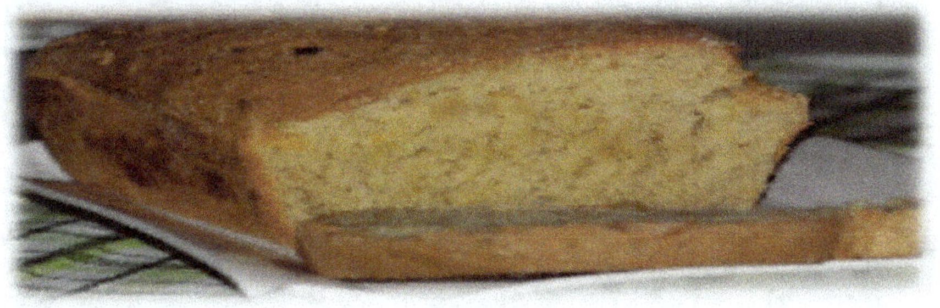

# Rutabaga and Onion Gratin

***Ingredients:***

- ✓ 2 lbs. rutabagas, peeled and thinly sliced
- ✓ 2 large onions, thinly sliced
- ✓ 1 cup of coconut milk
- ✓ 2 cloves garlic, minced
- ✓ 2 tbsp. nutritional yeast
- ✓ 2 tbsp. olive oil
- ✓ 1 tbsp. fresh thyme leaves
- ✓ Salt and pepper to taste

***Preparation:***

1. Preheat the oven to 375°F (190°C).

2. In a large bowl, combine the rutabagas, onions, garlic, nutritional yeast, and thyme. Season with salt and pepper. Toss to combine.

3. Grease a baking dish with olive oil. Layer the rutabaga and onion mixture in the dish, alternating between the two and creating overlapping layers.

4. Once all the vegetables are layered, pour the coconut milk over the top.

5. Bake for 45 minutes with the dish covered with foil.

6. Remove the foil and bake for an additional 15-20 minutes, or until the top is golden and the vegetables are tender.

<u>***Nutritional Value (per serving):***</u> Calories: 200, Fat: 10g, Carbohydrates: 25g, Fiber: 6g, Protein: 3g, Sugar: 10g, Sodium: 300mg.

<u>***Prep Time:***</u> 1 hour

**N**ote: This Rutabaga and Onion Gratin recipe is a delicious and nutritious dinner option that is suitable for the Candida diet. It is gluten-free, sugar-free, and packed with healthy fats, fiber, and essential nutrients.

# *Lemon Chicken*

<u>***Ingredients:***</u>

- ✓ 4 boneless, skinless chicken breasts
- ✓ 2 tablespoons of olive oil
- ✓ 2 cloves of garlic, minced
- ✓ 1 teaspoon of dried oregano
- ✓ 1 teaspoon of dried basil
- ✓ 1/2 teaspoon of salt
- ✓ 1/4 teaspoon of black pepper
- ✓ 1/2 cup of chicken broth
- ✓ Juice of 1 lemon
- ✓ Fresh parsley for garnish (optional)

<u>***Preparation:***</u>

1. Start by coating the chicken breasts with salt and pepper on both sides.
2. Heat the olive oil in a large pan over average-high heat.

3. Add the chicken breasts and cook for 6-7 minutes per side, or until no longer pink in the center.
4. After taking it out of the skillet, set the chicken aside.
5. In the same pan, combine the minced garlic, dried oregano, and dried basil.
6. Cook for approximately one minute, or until aromatic.
7. Add the lemon juice and chicken stock to the skillet. Stir to mix.
8. Return the chicken to the skillet and let it simmer in the sauce for 2-3 minutes.
9. Garnish with fresh parsley before serving.

**_Nutritional Value (per serving):_** Calories: 250, Fat: 10g, Carbohydrates: 2g, Fiber: 1g, Protein: 35g, Sugar: 1g, Sodium: 400mg.

**_Prep Time:_** 20 minutes

**N**ote: This lemon chicken recipe is a delicious and nutritious dinner option that is suitable for the Candida diet. It is gluten-free, sugar-free, and packed with healthy fats, fiber, and essential nutrients.

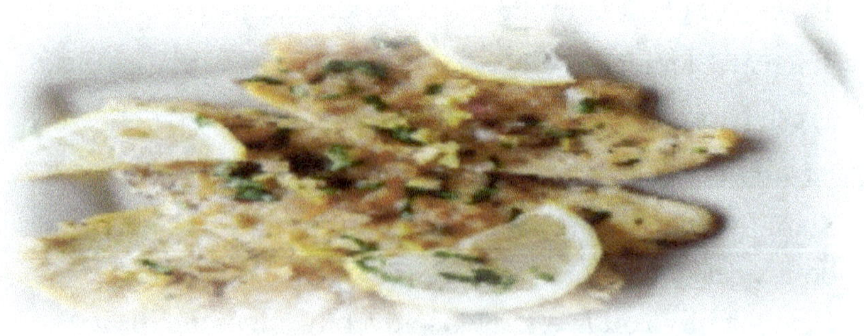

# Salmon Stew

**_Ingredients:_**

- ✓ 1 lb. wild-caught salmon fillet, cut into bite-sized pieces
- ✓ 1 tbsp. coconut oil
- ✓ 1 onion, chopped
- ✓ 2 garlic cloves, minced
- ✓ 1 red bell pepper, chopped
- ✓ 1 green bell pepper, chopped
- ✓ 1 can (14 oz.) unsweetened coconut milk
- ✓ 1 tbsp. fresh lime juice
- ✓ Salt and pepper to taste
- ✓ Fresh cilantro and tomato wedges for garnish

**_Preparation:_**

1. In a large saucepan, melt the coconut oil over medium heat.
2. Sauté the chopped onion and garlic until the onions are transparent.
3. Sauté the chopped red and green bell peppers for a further 5 minutes.
4. Pour in the unsweetened coconut milk and heat to a boil.
5. Add the salmon chunks, then reduce the heat to medium-low and cook, covered, for 6 to 8 minutes.
6. Season to taste with salt and pepper after adding the fresh lime juice.

7. Garnish the stew with tomato wedges and coarsely chopped fresh cilantro. Serve with lime wedges.

***Nutritional Value (per serving):*** Calories: 300, Fat: 20g, Carbohydrates: 8g, Fiber: 2g, Protein: 25g, Sugar: 3g, Sodium: 300mg.

***Prep Time:*** 30 minutes

**N**ote: This salmon stew recipe is a delicious and nutritious dinner option that is suitable for the Candida diet. It is gluten-free, sugar-free, and packed with healthy fats, fiber, and essential nutrients.

# Tandoori Chicken

### Ingredients:

✓ 4 boneless, skinless chicken breasts

✓ 1/2 cup full-fat coconut milk

✓ 2 tablespoons of olive oil

✓ 1 tablespoon of fresh lemon juice

✓ 1 tablespoon of paprika

✓ 1 tablespoon of ground cumin

✓ 1 tablespoon of ground coriander

✓ 1 teaspoon of ground turmeric

✓ 1/2 teaspoon of ground cinnamon

✓ 1/2 teaspoon of ground ginger

✓ 1/2 teaspoon of cayenne pepper

✓ Salt and pepper to taste

✓ Fresh cilantro for garnish

Preparation:

1. Start by covering the chicken breasts with salt and pepper on both sides.
2. In a large bowl, whisk together the coconut milk, olive oil, lemon juice, paprika, cumin, coriander, turmeric, cinnamon, ginger, cayenne pepper, salt, and pepper.
3. Add the chicken breasts to the bowl and toss to coat them in the marinade.
4. Cover the bowl with plastic wrap and chill for at least 2 hours, preferably overnight.
5. Preheat the oven to 400°F (200°C).
6. Place the chicken breasts on a parchment-lined baking pan.
7. Bake for 20–25 minutes, or until the chicken is done and no longer pink in the center.
8. Garnish with fresh cilantro before serving.

***Nutritional Value (per serving):*** Calories: 250, Fat: 12g, Carbohydrates: 4g, Fiber: 1g, Protein: 32g, Sugar: 1g, Sodium: 300mg.

***Prep Time (including marinating time:*** 2 hour, 30 minutes

**N**ote: This Tandoori Chicken recipe is a delicious and nutritious dinner option that is suitable for the Candida diet. It is gluten-free, sugar-free, and packed with healthy fats, fiber, and essential nutrients.

# Artichoke Salad With Coconut Balsamic Vinaigrette

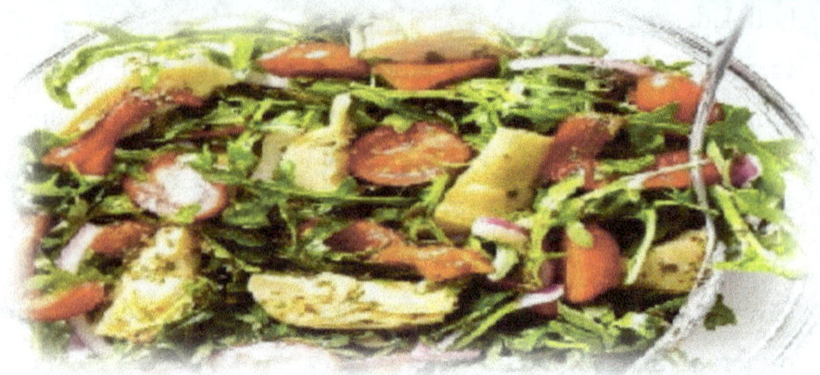

### *Ingredients:*

- ✓ 1 can of drained and washed artichoke hearts.
- ✓ 1 cup of mixed greens
- ✓ 1/2 cup of cherry tomatoes, halved
- ✓ 1/4 cup of toasted, sliced almonds
- ✓ 1/4 cup of coconut balsamic vinaigrette (see recipe below)

### *Coconut Balsamic Vinaigrette Ingredients:*

- ✓ 1/2 cup extra virgin olive oil
- ✓ 1/4 cup apple cider vinegar
- ✓ 2 tablespoons of coconut aminos
- ✓ 1 clove of garlic, minced
- ✓ 1 teaspoon of mustard powder
- ✓ Salt and pepper to taste
- ✓ 1 sprig of fresh rosemary

## Preparation:

1. In a large bowl, combine the mixed greens, artichoke hearts, and cherry tomatoes.
2. Drizzle the salad with 4 to 6 tablespoons of the coconut balsamic vinaigrette and gently toss to coat.
3. Sprinkle the salad with toasted, sliced almonds.

## Coconut Balsamic Vinaigrette Preparation:

1. In a container with a lid, whisk together the extra virgin olive oil, apple cider vinegar, coconut aminos, minced garlic, and mustard powder.
2. Season with salt and pepper to taste, then cover and shake thoroughly.
3. Add the sprig of fresh rosemary to the container.
4. Cover the container and let the vinaigrette sit at room temperature for at least 30 minutes, or until the flavors have developed.

**Nutritional Value (per serving):** Calories: 300, Fat: 20g, Carbohydrates: 8g, Fiber: 2g, Protein: 10g, Sugar: 1g, Sodium: 300mg.

**Prep Time:** 15 minutes

Note: This Artichoke Salad with Coconut Balsamic Vinaigrette recipe is a delicious and nutritious dinner option that is suitable for the Candida diet. It is gluten-free, sugar-free, and packed with healthy fats, fiber, and essential nutrients.

# Sheet-Pan Chicken

### Ingredients:

- ✓ 4 boneless, skinless chicken breasts
- ✓ 1 cup of red onion wedges
- ✓ 1 Granny Smith apple, cut into wedges
- ✓ 1 cup canned coconut milk
- ✓ 1 teaspoon of mustard powder
- ✓ 1 teaspoon of mustard seeds
- ✓ Fresh, chopped parsley for garnish
- ✓ Salt and pepper to taste

### Preparation:

1. Preheat the oven to 425°F (218°C).
2. Drizzle 1 tablespoon of oil over a rimmed sheet pan.
3. Season both sides of the chicken breasts with salt and pepper.
4. Place the chicken breasts on the prepared sheet pan and roast for 15 minutes.
5. Remove the pan from the oven and nestle the red onion wedges and Granny Smith apple wedges around the chicken.
6. In a small bowl, whisk together the canned coconut milk, mustard powder, and mustard seeds.
7. Drizzle the coconut milk mixture over the vegetables and chicken.

8. Return the sheet pan to the oven and roast for an additional 10 minutes, until the coconut milk mixture has reduced and the edges of the cabbage wedges have browned.

9. Garnish with freshly cut parsley and serve immediately.

***Nutritional Value (per serving):*** Calories: 300, Fat: 12g, Carbohydrates: 10g, Fiber: 2g, Protein: 32g, Sugar: 1g, Sodium: 300mg.

***Prep Time:*** 35 minutes

**N**ote: This sheet pan chicken recipe is a delicious and nutritious dinner option that is suitable for the Candida diet. It is gluten-free, sugar-free, and packed with healthy fats, fiber, and essential nutrients.

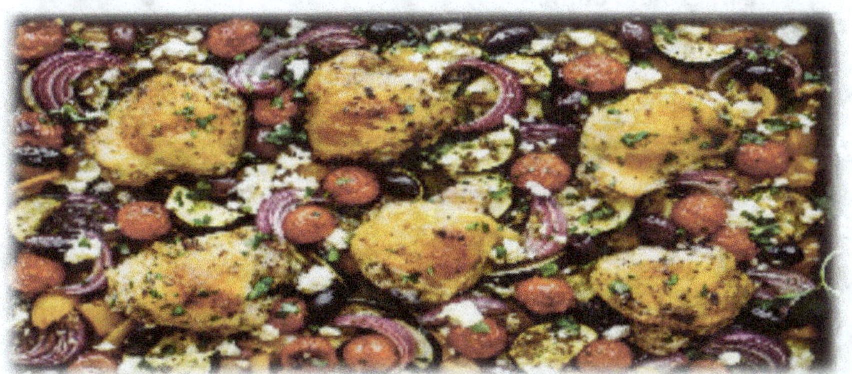

## Spicy Jalapeno Meatballs

***Ingredients:***

✓  1 Tbsp. oil, olive, or coconut

✓  1 lb. ground chicken or turkey

- ✓ 1/4 cup cilantro, finely minced
- ✓ 1 jalapeno, finely minced
- ✓ 1/4 cup almond flour
- ✓ 1/4 cup coconut flour
- ✓ 1/2 tsp. baking soda
- ✓ 1/2 tsp. salt
- ✓ 1/4 tsp. black pepper
- ✓ 1/2 tsp. garlic powder
- ✓ 1/2 tsp. onion powder
- ✓ 1/2 tsp. paprika
- ✓ 1/4 tsp. cayenne pepper
- ✓ 1/4 tsp. ground cumin
- ✓ 1/4 tsp. dried oregano
- ✓ 1/4 tsp. dried thyme

### ***Preparation:***

1. Preheat the oven to 400°F.
2. In a large bowl, combine the ground chicken or turkey, cilantro, jalapeno, almond flour, coconut flour, baking soda, salt, black pepper, garlic powder, onion powder, paprika, cayenne pepper, cumin, oregano, and thyme. Mix until well combined.
3. Form the mixture into meatballs and set them on a baking pan.
4. Bake for 20 to 25 minutes, or until the meatballs are well cooked.

<u>*Nutritional Value (per serving):*</u> Calories: 250, Fat: 15g, Carbohydrates: 5g, Fiber: 2g, Protein: 25g, Sugar: 1g, Sodium: 400mg.

<u>*Prep Time:*</u> 30 minutes

**N**ote: This spicy jalapeno meatball recipe is a delicious and nutritious dinner option that is suitable for the Candida diet. It is gluten-free, sugar-free, and packed with healthy fats, fiber, and essential nutrients.

# Grilled Chicken With Roasted Vegetables

## <u>*Ingredients:*</u>

- ✓ 2 boneless, skinless chicken breasts
- ✓ 1 red bell pepper, sliced
- ✓ 1 yellow bell pepper, sliced
- ✓ 1 zucchini, sliced
- ✓ 1 yellow squash, sliced
- ✓ 1/2 onion, sliced
- ✓ 2 garlic cloves, minced
- ✓ 2 tbsp. olive oil
- ✓ Salt and pepper to taste

## <u>*Preparation:*</u>

1. Preheat the grill to medium-high heat.

2. In a large bowl, toss the sliced bell peppers, sliced zucchini, sliced yellow squash, sliced onion, minced garlic, olive oil, salt, and pepper until evenly coated.

3. Place the vegetables on a baking sheet in a single layer.

4. Place the chicken breasts on the vegetables.

5. Add salt and pepper to the chicken breasts as desired.

6. Grill the chicken and vegetables for 10–12 minutes on each side, or until the chicken is cooked through and the vegetables are tender and golden brown.

**_Nutritional Value (per serving):_** Calories: 300, Fat: 14g, Carbohydrates: 10g, Fiber: 3g, Protein: 35, Sugar: 5g, Sodium: 200mg.

**_Prep Time:_** 30 minutes

**N**ote: This Grilled Chicken with Roasted Vegetables recipe is a delicious and nutritious dinner option that is suitable for the Candida diet. It is gluten-free, sugar-free, and packed with protein, fiber, and essential nutrients.

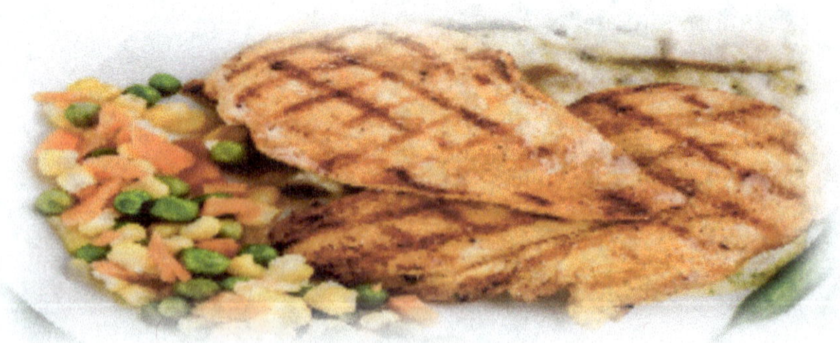

# CHAPTER 4

## CANDIDA-FRIENDLY SNACKS AND DESSERTS RECIPES FOR SUSTENANCE

### Sliced Cucumber With Homemade Chunky Guacamole

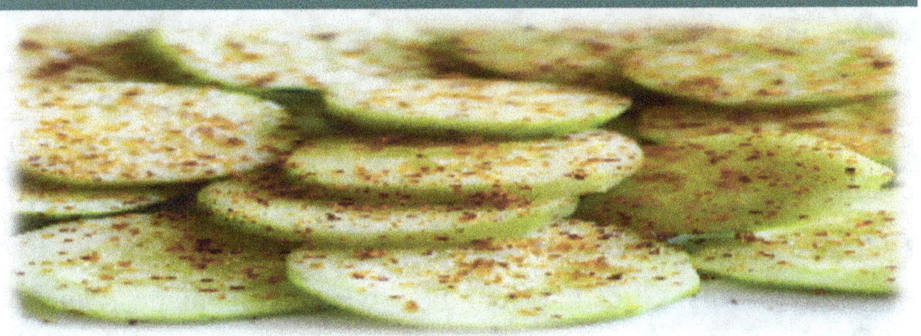

**_Ingredients:_**

- ✓ 2 medium-ripe avocados, peeled, pitted, and diced
- ✓ 1/4 cup finely chopped red onion
- ✓ 1/2 large tomato, diced
- ✓ 1/4 cup chopped fresh cilantro
- ✓ 1 tablespoon of fresh lime juice
- ✓ 1/2 teaspoon salt, or to taste
- ✓ 1/4 teaspoon black pepper, or to taste
- ✓ 2 medium cucumbers, sliced

<u>*Preparation:*</u>

1. In a medium bowl, combine the diced avocados, chopped red onion, diced tomato, chopped cilantro, lime juice, salt, and black pepper.
2. Gently mash the ingredients together with a fork until the desired consistency is reached.
3. Place the guacamole in a serving dish and garnish with additional cilantro and a lime wedge, if desired.
4. Serve the homemade chunky guacamole with the sliced cucumbers for dipping.

Nutritional Value (per serving):, Calories: 150, Fat: 13g, Carbohydrates: 10g, Fiber: 7g, Protein: 2g, Sugar: 2g, Sodium: 300mg.

<u>*Prep Time:*</u> 15 minutes

**N**ote: This Sliced Cucumber with Homemade Chunky Guacamole recipe is a delicious and nutritious snack option that is suitable for the Candida diet. It is gluten-free, sugar-free, and packed with healthy fats, fiber, and essential nutrients.

# Hard-Boiled Eggs

<u>*Ingredients:*</u>

✓  4 large eggs
✓  Salt and pepper to taste

<u>*Preparation:*</u>

1. Put the eggs in a pot and cover it with cold water.

2.  Bring the water to a boil over high heat.

3.  Once the water has boiled, remove the pot from the heat and cover it with a lid.

4.  Allow the eggs to rest in the heated water for 10–12 minutes.

5.  After 10–12 minutes, remove the eggs from the hot water and place them in a bowl of ice water to cool.

6.  Once the eggs are cool, peel them and slice them in half.

7.  Season the hard-boiled eggs with salt and pepper to taste.

***Nutritional Value (per serving):*** Calories: 70, Fat: 5g, Protein: 6g, Sodium: 70mg.

***Prep Time:*** 15 minutes

**N**ote: This hard-boiled egg recipe is a simple and nutritious snack option that is suitable for the Candida diet. It is gluten-free, sugar-free, and packed with healthy fats, protein, and essential nutrients.

# Baked Chicken Drumsticks

***Ingredients:***

✓  4 chicken drumsticks
✓  1 tablespoon of olive oil
✓  1/2 teaspoon of garlic powder
✓  1/2 teaspoon of onion powder
✓  1/2 teaspoon of paprika
✓  1/4 teaspoon of dried oregano
✓  1/4 teaspoon of dried thyme
✓  Salt and pepper to taste

***Preparation:***

1.  Preheat the oven to 425°F.
2.  In a small bowl, combine the olive oil, garlic powder, onion powder, paprika, dried oregano, dried thyme, salt, and pepper.
3.  Use a paper towel to dry the chicken drumsticks.
4.  Brush the drumsticks with the oil and spice mixture, coating them evenly.
5.  Put the drumsticks on a baking sheet coated with parchment paper.
6.  Bake for 35–45 minutes, or until the chicken is golden brown and reaches an internal temperature of 165°F.

Nutritional Value (per serving): Calories: 220, Fat: 15g, Protein: 20g, Sodium: 400mg.

***Prep Time:*** 10 minutes plus baking time

**N**ote: This Baked Chicken Drumsticks recipe is a delicious and nutritious snack or dessert option that is suitable for the Candida diet. It is gluten-free, sugar-free, and packed with healthy fats, protein, and essential nutrients.

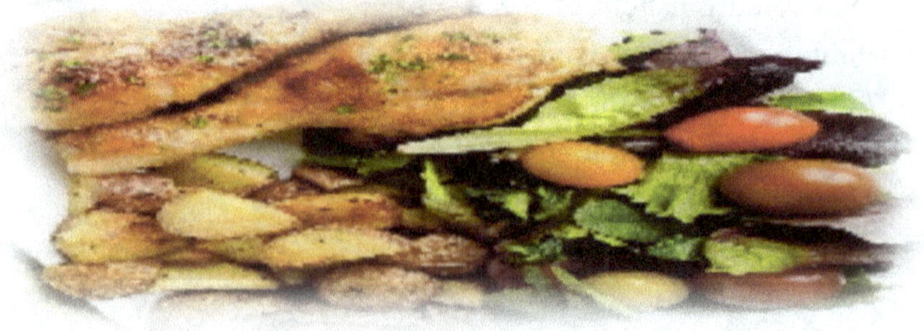

# Coconut Flour Chocolate Chip Cookies

**Ingredients:**

- ✓ 1/2 cup coconut flour
- ✓ 1/4 cup coconut oil, melted
- ✓ 1/4 cup monk fruit sweetener
- ✓ 2 eggs
- ✓ 1 tsp. vanilla extract
- ✓ 1/2 teaspoon baking powder
- ✓ 1/4 tsp. salt
- ✓ 1/4 cup sugar-free chocolate chips

**Preparation:**

1. Preheat the oven to 350°F.
2. In a large bowl, whisk together the coconut flour, monk fruit sweetener, baking powder, and salt.
3. In a separate dish, combine the melted coconut oil, eggs, and vanilla essence.
4. Add the wet components to the dry ingredients and mix thoroughly.
5. Fold in the sugar-free chocolate chips.
6. Using a cookie scoop or spoon, drop the dough onto a baking sheet lined with parchment paper.
7. Bake the cookies for 12 to 15 minutes, or until golden brown.

8. Let the cookies cool on the baking sheet for 5 minutes before transferring them to a wire rack to complete cooling.

Nutritional Value (per serving): Calories: 90, Fat: 7g, Carbohydrates: 5g, Fiber: 3g, Protein: 2g, Sugar: 1g, Sodium: 70mg.

***Prep Time:*** 15 minutes plus baking time

**N**ote: This Coconut Flour Chocolate Chip Cookies recipe is a delicious and nutritious snack or dessert option that is suitable for the Candida diet. It is gluten-free, sugar-free, and packed with healthy fats, fiber, and essential nutrients.

# *Vanilla Coconut Macaroons*

***Ingredients:***

✓ 3 cups unsweetened shredded coconut

✓ 3/4 cup sweetened condensed milk

✓ 1 1/2 teaspoons of vanilla extract

✓ 1/4 teaspoon salt

✓ 1/2 cup semisweet chocolate chips (optional)

***Preparation:***

1. Preheat the oven to 350°F (175°C).

2. Put parchment paper on a baking pan.

3. In a large bowl, combine the shredded coconut, sweetened condensed milk, vanilla extract, and salt. Stir until well combined.

4. Use a small cookie scoop to form the mixture into mounds and place them on the prepared baking sheet.

5. Bake for 10–12 minutes, or until the macaroons are golden brown around the edges.

6. If using chocolate, melt the chocolate chips in the microwave in 20-second intervals, stirring between each interval.

7. Sprinkle the melted chocolate over the chilled macaroons.

***Nutritional Value (per serving):*** Calories: 110, Fat: 7g, Carbohydrates: 11g, Fiber: 2g, Protein: 1g, Sugar: 9g, Sodium: 80mg.

***Prep Time:*** 20 minutes plus baking time

Note: This Vanilla Coconut Macaroons recipe is a delicious and nutritious snack or dessert option that is suitable for the Candida diet. It is gluten-free, sugar-free, and packed with healthy fats, fiber, and essential nutrients.

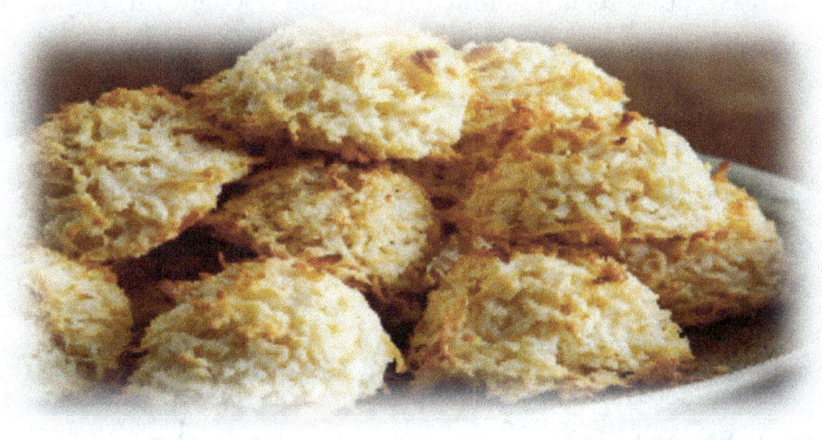

# Raspberry Pie Cookies

**_Ingredients:_**

- ✓ 1/2 cup coconut flour
- ✓ 1/4 cup coconut oil, melted
- ✓ 1/4 cup monk fruit sweetener
- ✓ 2 eggs
- ✓ 1 tsp. vanilla extract
- ✓ 1/2 teaspoon baking powder
- ✓ 1/4 tsp. salt
- ✓ 1/4 cup fresh raspberries, mashed

**_Preparation:_**

1. Preheat the oven to 350°F.
2. In a large bowl, whisk together the coconut flour, monk fruit sweetener, baking powder, and salt.
3. In a separate dish, combine the melted coconut oil, eggs, and vanilla essence.
4. Add the wet components to the dry ingredients and mix thoroughly.
5. Fold in the crushed raspberries.
6. Using a cookie scoop or spoon, transfer the dough to a baking sheet coated with parchment.
7. Bake the cookies for 12–15 minutes, or until golden brown.
8. Let the cookies cool on the baking sheet for 5 minutes before transferring them to a wire rack to complete cooling.

<u>*Nutritional Value (per serving): Calories:*</u> 90, Fat: 7g, Carbohydrates: 5g, Fiber: 3g, Protein: 2g, Sugar: 1g, Sodium: 70mg.

<u>*Prep Time:*</u> 20 minutes plus baking time

**N**ote: This Raspberry Pie Cookies recipe is a delicious and nutritious snack or dessert option that is suitable for the Candida diet. It is gluten-free, sugar-free, and packed with healthy fats, fiber, and essential nutrients.

# Blueberry Panna Cotta

<u>*Ingredients:*</u>

- ✓ 1 cup of frozen blueberries
- ✓ 1/4 cup of water
- ✓ 1/4 tsp. powdered stevia
- ✓ 1/2 tsp. agar powder
- ✓ 1 1/2 cups almond milk
- ✓ 1/4 tsp. vanilla extract

<u>*Preparation:*</u>

1. In a small saucepan over average heat, combine the frozen blueberries, water, stevia, and agar agar powder.

2. Bring the blueberry mixture to a boil, stirring regularly, then immediately remove from heat.

3. Cool for 10 to 15 minutes, then spoon equal amounts of the blueberry mixture into ramekins or small serving glasses.

4. Refrigerate until firm, about 2 to 4 hours.

5. In another saucepan, heat the almond milk and vanilla extract over medium heat until it begins to simmer.

6. Pour equal portions of the milk mixture into ramekins or small serving glasses.

7. Refrigerate until firm, about 2 to 4 hours.

8. Once the milk layer is set, spoon equal amounts of the blueberry mixture on top of the chilled panna cottas.

9. Chill until firm, about 1 hour.

10. Garnish with fresh blueberries and mint, and serve.

***Nutritional Value (per serving): Calories:*** 70, Fat: 3g, Carbohydrates: 10g, Fiber: 2g, Protein: 1g, Sugar: 6g, Sodium: 80mg.

***Prep Time:*** 20 minutes plus baking time

**N**ote: This Blueberry Panna Cotta recipe is a delicious and nutritious snack or dessert option that is suitable for the Candida diet. It is gluten-free, sugar-free, and packed with healthy fats, fiber, and essential nutrients.

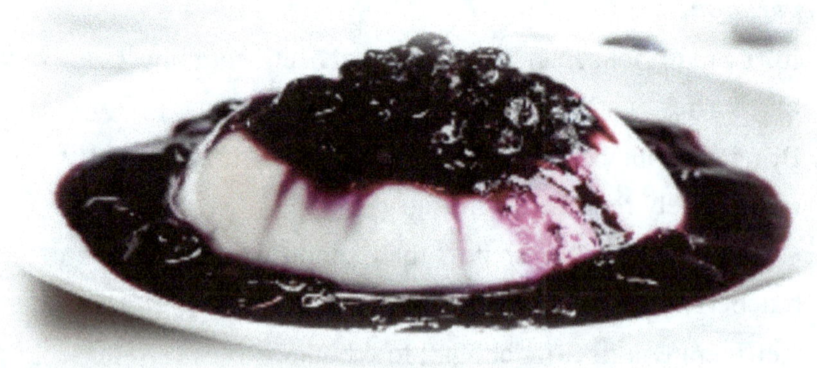

# Lemon Coconut Cookies

**_Ingredients:_**

- ✓ 1 cup unsweetened, shredded coconut
- ✓ 1/4 cup coconut flour
- ✓ 1/4 cup coconut oil, melted
- ✓ 1/4 cup of lemon juice
- ✓ 1/4 cup monk fruit sweetener
- ✓ 1/4 cup almond milk
- ✓ 1 tsp. vanilla extract
- ✓ 1/4 tsp. baking powder
- ✓ 1/4 tsp. salt

**_Preparation:_**

1. Preheat the oven to 350°F (175°C).
2. In a large bowl, combine the shredded coconut, coconut flour, melted coconut oil, lemon juice, monk fruit sweetener, almond milk, vanilla extract, baking powder, and salt.
3. Mix until the ingredients are completely mixed.
4. Using a cookie scoop or spoon, roll the dough into tiny balls and lay them on a baking sheet coated with parchment.
5. Bake the cookies for 12–15 minutes, or until golden brown.
6. Let the cookies cool on the baking sheet for 5 minutes before transferring them to a wire rack to complete cooling.

<u>***Nutritional Value (per serving):Calories:***</u> 80, Fat: 6g, Carbohydrates: 5g, Fiber: 2g, Protein: 1g, Sugar: 1g, Sodium: 60mg.

<u>***Prep Time:***</u> 20 minutes plus baking time

**N**ote: This Lemon Coconut Cookies recipe is a delicious and nutritious snack or dessert option that is suitable for the Candida diet. It is gluten-free, sugar-free, and packed with healthy fats, fiber, and essential nutrients.

# Strawberry Muffins

<u>***Ingredients:***</u>

- ✓ 1 cup of quinoa flour
- ✓ 1 cup light buckwheat flour
- ✓ 1 tsp. psyllium husk powder
- ✓ 1/4 cup coconut oil, melted
- ✓ 1 tsp. cinnamon
- ✓ 1/2 tsp. salt
- ✓ 1 tsp. baking powder
- ✓ 1 tsp. baking soda
- ✓ 1 cup fresh or frozen strawberries, diced
- ✓ 1/4 cup unsweetened applesauce
- ✓ 1/4 cup maple syrup
- ✓ 1/2 cup unsweetened almond milk
- ✓ 1 tsp. vanilla extract

*__Preparation:__*

1. Preheat the oven to 350°F (175°C). Line a 12-cup muffin pan with paper liners and set aside.
2. In a large mixing bowl, combine quinoa flour, light buckwheat flour, psyllium husk powder, cinnamon, salt, baking powder, and baking soda. Whisk to combine; set aside.
3. In another large bowl, add melted coconut oil, unsweetened applesauce, maple syrup, almond milk, and vanilla extract. Whisk to combine.
4. Add the wet ingredients to the dry ingredients and stir until just combined.
5. Gently fold in the diced strawberries.
6. Divide the mixture evenly between the muffin cups you've prepared.
7. Bake for 20–25 minutes, or until a toothpick inserted into the middle of a muffin comes out clean.
8. Allow the muffins to cool in the pan for 5 minutes before transferring them to a wire rack to cool fully.

*__Nutritional Value (per serving): Calories:__* 150, Fat: 5g, Carbohydrates: 23g, Fiber: 3g, Protein: 3g, Sugar: 4g, Sodium: 300mg.

*__Prep Time:__* 15 minutes plus baking time

**N**ote: This strawberry muffin recipe is a delicious and nutritious snack or dessert option that is suitable for the Candida diet. It is gluten-free, sugar-free, and packed with healthy fats, fiber, and essential nutrients.

# Low-Carb Cinnamon Rolls

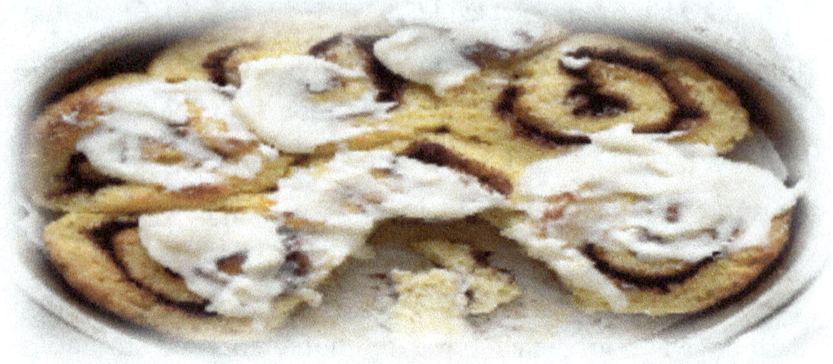

### *Ingredients:*

### *For the dough:*

- ✓ 1 cup of almond flour
- ✓ 1/4 cup coconut flour
- ✓ 1/4 cup psyllium husk powder
- ✓ 1/4 cup erythritol
- ✓ 1 tsp. baking powder
- ✓ 1/2 tsp. baking soda
- ✓ 1/4 tsp. salt
- ✓ 1/4 cup coconut oil, melted
- ✓ 1/4 cup unsweetened almond milk
- ✓ 2 large eggs

### *For the filling:*

- ✓ 1/4 cup coconut oil, melted

✓ 1/4 cup erythritol

✓ 2 tsp. ground cinnamon

***For the glaze:***

✓ 1/4 cup coconut butter, melted

✓ 2 Tbsp. unsweetened almond milk

✓ 1 Tbsp. erythritol

✓ 1/2 tsp. vanilla extract

***Preparation:***

1. Preheat the oven to 350°F (175°C). Line a baking sheet with parchment paper and set aside.

2. In a large bowl, add almond flour, coconut flour, psyllium husk powder, erythritol, baking powder, baking soda, and salt. Whisk to combine; set aside.

3. In another large bowl, add melted coconut oil, unsweetened almond milk, and eggs. Whisk to combine.

4. Add the wet ingredients to the dry ingredients and stir until just combined.

5. In a small bowl, mix together the melted coconut oil, erythritol, and cinnamon for the filling.

6. Roll out the dough between two sheets of parchment paper into a rectangle shape.

7. Spread the filling mixture evenly on the dough, leaving a little border around the edges.

8. Roll up the dough tightly, starting from the long side.

9. Cut the roll into 8 equal pieces and place them on the prepared baking sheet.

10. Bake for 20–25 minutes, or until the cinnamon rolls are golden brown.

11. In a small bowl, whisk together the melted coconut butter, unsweetened almond milk, erythritol, and vanilla extract for the glaze.

12. Drizzle the glaze over the cinnamon rolls and serve.

Nutritional Value (per serving): Calories: 280, Fat: 25g, Carbohydrates: 10g, Fiber: 7g, Protein: 7g, Sugar: 1g, Sodium: 250mg.

***Prep Time:*** 30 minutes plus baking time

**N**ote: This low-carb cinnamon roll recipe is a delicious and nutritious snack or dessert option that is suitable for the Candida diet. It is gluten-free, sugar-free, and packed with healthy fats, fiber, and essential nutrients.

# Low-Carb Enchiladas

***Ingredients:***

***For the filling:***

✓ 1 cup of shredded rotisserie chicken

✓ 1/4 cup canned black beans, drained and rinsed

✓ 1/4 cup canned corn, drained

✓ 1/4 cup diced red bell pepper

✓ 1/4 cup diced green bell pepper

- ✓ 1/4 cup diced onion
- ✓ 1/4 cup chopped fresh cilantro
- ✓ 1/4 cup of salsa
- ✓ 1/4 cup unsweetened almond milk
- ✓ 1 tsp. ground cumin
- ✓ 1 tsp. chili powder
- ✓ 1/2 tsp. garlic powder
- ✓ 1/2 tsp. onion powder
- ✓ Salt and pepper, to taste

***For the rolls:***
- ✓ 4 large eggs
- ✓ 1/4 cup unsweetened almond milk
- ✓ 1/4 cup coconut flour
- ✓ 1/4 cup psyllium husk powder
- ✓ 1/4 cup erythritol
- ✓ 1 tsp. baking powder
- ✓ 1/2 tsp. baking soda
- ✓ 1/4 tsp. salt

***For the sauce:***
- ✓ 1/4 cup unsweetened almond milk
- ✓ 1/4 cup canned pumpkin puree
- ✓ 1/4 cup of salsa
- ✓ 1 tsp. chili powder
- ✓ 1/2 tsp. garlic powder

✓ 1/2 tsp. onion powder

✓ Salt and pepper, to taste

### ***Preparation:***

1. Preheat the oven to 350°F (175°C). Line a baking sheet with parchment paper and set aside.

2. In a large bowl, mix together the shredded rotisserie chicken, black beans, corn, red bell pepper, green bell pepper, onion, cilantro, salsa, unsweetened almond milk, cumin, chili powder, garlic powder, onion powder, salt, and pepper for the filling.

3. In another large bowl, whisk together the eggs, unsweetened almond milk, coconut flour, psyllium husk powder, erythritol, baking powder, baking soda, and salt for the rolls.

4. In a small bowl, whisk together the unsweetened almond milk, canned pumpkin puree, salsa, chili powder, garlic powder, onion powder, salt, and pepper for the sauce.

5. Pour the sauce mixture into a small saucepan and heat over medium heat, stirring occasionally, until the sauce thickens, about 5 minutes.

6. Spread a thin layer of the sauce mixture on the parchment paper.

7. Spread a thin layer of the filling mixture on top of the sauce mixture.

8. Drop spoonfuls of the roll mixture onto the filling mixture, spreading it out evenly.

9.  Bake for 20–25 minutes, or until the rolls are golden brown and cooked through.

10. Serve the rolls with the remaining sauce mixture on top.

***Nutritional Value (per serving):*** Calories: 250, Fat: 15g, Carbohydrates: 15g, Fiber: 5g, Protein: 15g, Sugar: 1g, Sodium: 300mg.

***Prep Time:*** 30 minutes plus baking time

**N**ote: This low-carb enchilada roll recipe is a delicious and nutritious snack or dessert option that is suitable for the Candida diet. It is gluten-free, sugar-free, and packed with healthy fats, fiber, and essential nutrients.

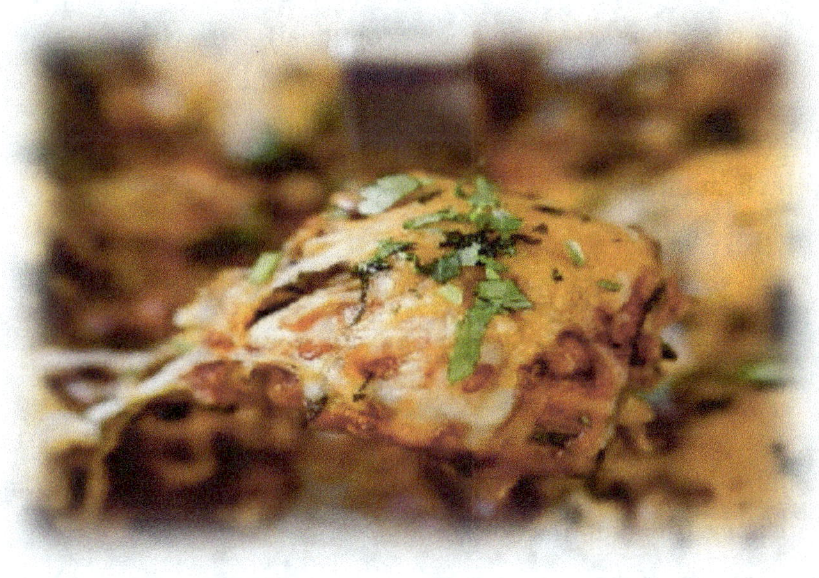

# Low-Carb "Potato" Gratin

### Ingredients:

- ✓ 1 large cauliflower head, cut into florets
- ✓ 1 cup of unsweetened almond milk
- ✓ 1 cup of vegetable broth
- ✓ 2 cloves garlic, minced
- ✓ 2 tbsp. nutritional yeast
- ✓ 1 tsp Dijon mustard
- ✓ 1/2 tsp. onion powder
- ✓ 1/2 tsp. thyme
- ✓ Salt and pepper to taste
- ✓ 1/4 cup shredded vegan cheese (optional)
- ✓ Fresh parsley, chopped (for garnish)

### Preparation:

1. Preheat the oven to 375°F (190°C).
2. Grease a baking dish.
3. Heat water in a big saucepan until it boils.
4. Add the cauliflower florets and cook for 5–6 minutes, until tender. Drain well.
5. In a blender, combine the almond milk, vegetable broth, garlic, nutritional yeast, Dijon mustard, onion powder, thyme, salt, and pepper. Blend until smooth.
6. Place the cooked cauliflower in the prepared baking dish. Pour the blended mixture over the cauliflower.

7.  If using, sprinkle the shredded vegan cheese on top.

8.  Bake for 25–30 minutes, until the top is golden and bubbly.

9.  Garnish with fresh parsley before serving.

***Nutritional Value (per serving):*** Calories: 120, Fat: 5g, Carbohydrates: 10g, Fiber: 5g, Protein: 8g, Sugar: 3g, Sodium: 400mg.

***Prep Time:*** 15 minutes plus baking time

**N**ote: This low-carb "potato" gratin recipe is a delicious and nutritious side dish that is suitable for the Candida diet. It is gluten-free, sugar-free, and packed with healthy fats, fiber, and essential nutrients.

## Raw Buckwheat Ricotta

***Ingredients:***

✓  100g (3.5oz) raw buckwheat groats, soaked

✓  100g (3.5oz) raw cashews, soaked

✓  Juice of half a lemon

✓  1/8 tsp. Himalayan salt

✓  2 tbsp. filtered water

***Preparation:***

1.  Soak the raw buckwheat groats and raw cashews for at least 4 hours or overnight.

2.  Rinse and drain the soaked buckwheat groats and cashews.

3. In a food processor or high-speed blender, combine the soaked buckwheat groats, soaked cashews, lemon juice, Himalayan salt, and filtered water.

4. Blend the mixture until smooth and creamy, scraping down the sides as needed.

5. Transfer the mixture to a bowl and use it as a dairy-free ricotta alternative in your favorite recipes.

Nutritional Value (per serving): Calories: 120, Fat: 7g, Carbohydrates: 10g, Fiber: 2g, Protein: 5g, Sugar: 1g, Sodium: 50mg.

***Prep Time:*** 15 minutes excluding the soaking time for the buckwheat groats and cashews.

**N**ote: This raw buckwheat ricotta recipe is a delicious and nutritious dairy-free alternative suitable for the Candida diet. It is gluten-free, sugar-free, and packed with healthy fats, fiber, and essential nutrients.

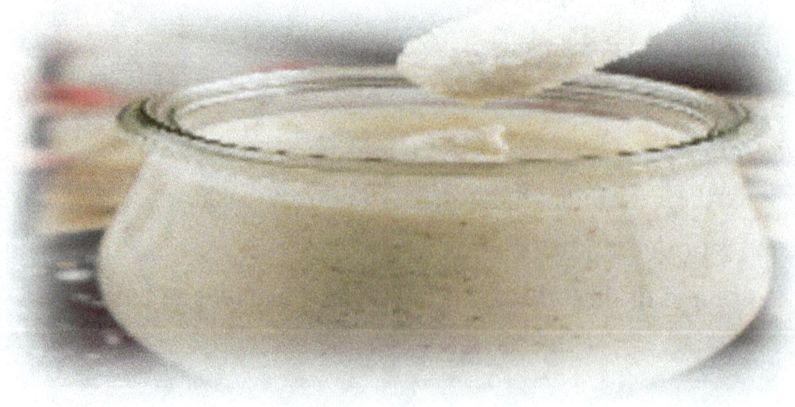

# Vegan Oatmeal Pancakes

## *Ingredients:*

- ✓ 200g (7oz) rolled oats
- ✓ 700g (24.7 oz) of filtered water
- ✓ Himalayan salt to taste (maximum ¼+⅛ tsp. for the Plantricious version)
- ✓ 2 tsp. baking powder
- ✓ 2 tsp. ground cinnamon
- ✓ 2 ripe bananas
- ✓ 2 tsp. apple cider vinegar
- ✓ 4 tbsp. ground flaxseeds
- ✓ 4 tbsp. water
- ✓ 2 tsp. vanilla extract
- ✓ Coconut oil for frying

## *Preparation:*

1. In a bowl, mix the ground flaxseeds with water and set aside for 5 minutes.
2. In a blender, process the rolled oats into flour.
3. Add water, salt, baking powder, ground cinnamon, bananas, apple cider vinegar, and vanilla extract to the blender. Blend until smooth.
4. Let the batter sit for 10 minutes.
5. Heat a non-stick frying pan over medium heat and add a small amount of coconut oil.

6. Pour 60 ml (1/4 cup) of batter into the pan for each pancake.

7. Cook until bubbles form on top of the pancake, then turn and cook until golden brown.

8. Continue with the remaining batter.

***Nutritional Value (per serving):*** Calories: 150, Fat: 3g, Carbohydrates: 25g, Fiber: 5g, Protein: 5g, Sugar: 5g, Sodium: 300mg.

***Prep Time:*** 20 minutes

**N**ote: These vegan oatmeal pancakes are a delicious and nutritious breakfast option that is suitable for the Candida diet. They are gluten-free, sugar-free, and packed with healthy fats, fiber, and essential nutrients. The preparation time for this recipe is about 20 minutes.

# Savory Sorghum Muffins

## *Ingredients:*

✓ 1 cup of sorghum flour

✓ 1/2 cup almond flour

✓ 1/2 cup tapioca flour

✓ 1 tsp. baking powder

✓ 1/2 tsp. baking soda

✓ 1/2 tsp. Himalayan salt

✓ 1/2 tsp. dried thyme

✓ 1/2 tsp. dried rosemary

✓ 1/2 tsp. garlic powder

✓ 1/2 tsp. onion powder

✓ 1/2 cup unsweetened almond milk

✓ 1/4 cup olive oil

✓ 2 tbsp. apple cider vinegar

✓ 2 tbsp. nutritional yeast

✓ 1/4 cup chopped fresh parsley

✓ 1/4 cup chopped fresh chives

***Preparation:***

1. Preheat the oven to 375°F (190°C).

2. Grease the muffin tray or set it with muffin cups.

3. In a large bowl, whisk together the sorghum flour, almond flour, tapioca flour, baking powder, baking soda, Himalayan salt, dried thyme, dried rosemary, garlic powder, and onion powder.

4. In a separate bowl, whisk together the almond milk, olive oil, apple cider vinegar, and nutritional yeast.

5. Add the wet ingredients to the dry ingredients and stir until just combined.

6. Fold in the chopped parsley and chives.

7. Spoon the mixture into the muffin cups, filling them approximately 3/4 full.

8. Bake the muffins for 20–25 minutes, or until golden brown and a toothpick inserted in the center comes out clean.

9. Allow the muffins to cool for a few minutes before removing them from the pan.

Nutritional Value (per serving): Calories: 150, Fat: 8g, Carbohydrates: 16g, Fiber: 2g, Protein: 4g, Sodium: 250mg.

**_Prep Time:_** 30 minutes plus baking time

**N**otte: These savory sorghum muffins are a delicious and nutritious snack or breakfast option that is suitable for the Candida diet. They are gluten-free, sugar-free, and packed with healthy fats, fiber, and essential nutrients.

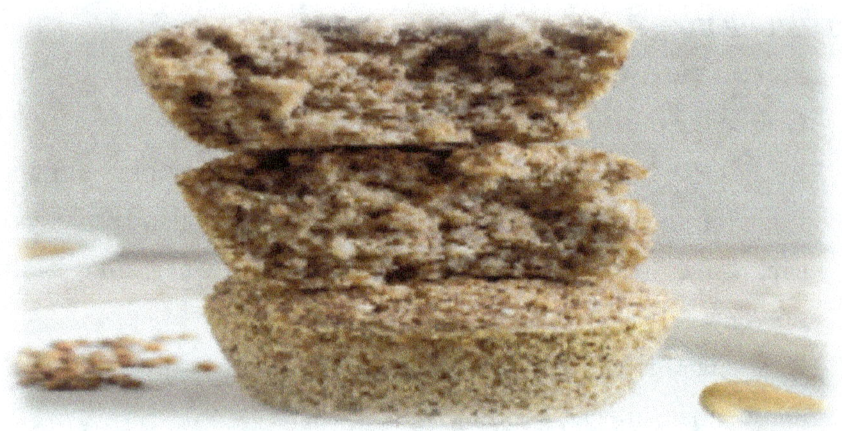

# Sprouted Buckwheat Crackers

**_Ingredients:_**

- ✓ 1 cup raw buckwheat groats
- ✓ 1/4 cup ground flaxseeds
- ✓ 1/4 cup chia seeds
- ✓ 1/4 cup sunflower seeds
- ✓ 1/4 cup pumpkin seeds
- ✓ 1/2 teaspoon sea salt

✓  1/2 teaspoon garlic powder

✓  1/2 teaspoon onion powder

✓  1/2 teaspoon dried rosemary

✓  1/2 teaspoon dried thyme

✓  1 cup of water

## ***Preparation:***

1.  Place the raw buckwheat groats in a large bowl and cover with water.

2.  Allow them to soak for at least 6 hours, preferably overnight.

3.  After soaking, rinse the buckwheat groats well and drain.

4.  In a large mixing bowl, combine the soaked buckwheat groats, ground flaxseeds, chia seeds, sunflower seeds, pumpkin seeds, sea salt, garlic powder, onion powder, dried rosemary, and dried thyme.

5.  Add 1 cup of water to the mixture and stir well until everything is combined. The mixture will be thick and should be spreadable.

6.  Preheat the oven to 170°C (340°F).

7.  Line a baking tray with baking paper, and spread the mixture thinly and as evenly as possible. You can use an additional sheet of baking paper to help you with that.

8.  Using a knife, score the crackers into the desired size and shape.

9. Bake for 30 minutes, then remove from the oven and carefully flip the crackers over. Peel off the baking paper and return to the oven for a further 20–30 minutes, or until the crackers are golden and crisp.

10. Allow the crackers to cool completely before breaking them along the scored lines.

___**Nutritional Value (per serving):**___ Calories: 120,Fat: 6g, Carbohydrates: 12g, Fiber: 3g, Protein: 4g, Sodium: 120mg.

___**Prep Time:**___ 30 minutes, including soaking and baking time.

**N**ote: These sprouted buckwheat crackers are a delicious and nutritious snack that is suitable for the Candida diet. They are gluten-free, sugar-free, and packed with healthy fats, fiber, and essential nutrients.

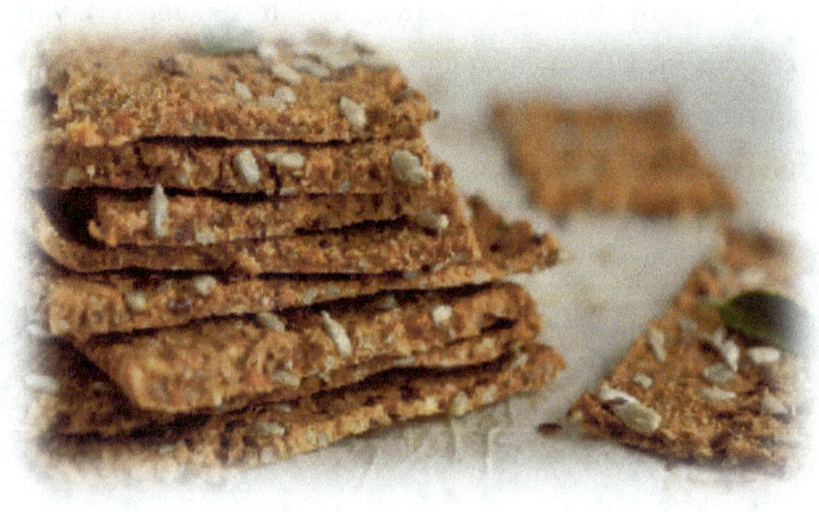

# CHAPTER 5
## *14-DAY MEAL PLAN FOR CANDIDA-FRIENDLY RECIPES*

### <u>Day 1</u>

* **Breakfast:** Vegan protein smoothie with almond milk, spinach, and chia seeds

* **Snack:** raw veggies with hummus

* **Lunch:** Grilled chicken with mixed greens salad and sugar-free balsamic vinaigrette

* **Snack:** sugar-free coconut milk yogurt with mixed berries

* **Dinner:** Baked salmon with roasted asparagus and quinoa

### <u>Day 2</u>

* **Breakfast:** Vegan oatmeal pancakes with blueberries and sugar-free maple syrup

* **Snack:** Carrot sticks with hummus

* **Lunch:** lentil soup with a side salad

* **Snack:** sugar-free coconut yogurt with mixed berries

* **Dinner:** Grilled chicken with roasted Brussels sprouts and sweet potatoes

### <u>Day 3</u>

* **Breakfast:** Scrambled eggs with spinach and mushrooms

* **Snack:** sugar-free almond milk latte

* **Lunch:** Tuna salad with mixed greens and sugar-free ranch dressing

* **Snack:** sugar-free coconut milk yogurt with chia seeds

* **Dinner:** Grilled shrimp, zucchini noodles, and tomato sauce

## Day 4

* **Breakfast:** Vegan protein smoothie with almond milk, spinach, and chia seeds

* **Snack:** Raw veggies with guacamole

* **Lunch:** Chicken salad with mixed greens and sugar-free balsamic vinaigrette

* **Snack:** sugar-free coconut milk yogurt with mixed berries

* **Dinner:** Baked chicken with roasted broccoli and cauliflower rice

## Day 5

* **Breakfast:** Vegan protein pancakes with sugar-free maple syrup and mixed berries

* **Snack:** A sugar-free protein bar

* **Lunch:** Turkey chili with mixed green salad

* **Snack:** Sugar-free coconut milk yogurt with sliced almonds

* **Dinner:** Grilled steak with roasted sweet potato and green beans

# Day 6

* **Breakfast:** Vegan protein smoothie with almond milk, spinach, and chia seeds

* **Snack:** raw veggies with hummus

* **Lunch:** Grilled chicken with mixed greens salad and sugar-free balsamic vinaigrette

* **Snack:** sugar-free coconut milk yogurt with mixed berries

* **Dinner:** baked salmon, roasted Brussels sprouts, and quinoa

# Day 7

* **Breakfast:** Scrambled eggs with spinach and mushrooms

* **Snack:** sugar-free almond milk latte

* **Lunch:** Tuna salad with mixed greens and sugar-free ranch dressing

* **Snack:** sugar-free coconut milk yogurt with chia seeds

* Dinner: Grilled shrimp, zucchini noodles, and tomato sauce

# Day 8

* **Breakfast:** Vegan protein smoothie with almond milk, spinach, and chia seeds

* **Snack:** Raw veggies with guacamole

- ★ **Lunch:** Chicken salad with mixed greens and sugar-free balsamic vinaigrette

- ★ **Snack:** sugar-free coconut milk yogurt with mixed berries

- ★ **Dinner:** Baked chicken with roasted broccoli and cauliflower rice

## Day 9

- ★ **Breakfast:** Vegan oatmeal pancakes with blueberries and sugar-free maple syrup

- ★ **Snack:** Carrot sticks with hummus

- ★ **Lunch:** lentil soup with a side salad

- ★ **Snack:** sugar-free coconut yogurt with mixed berries

- ★ **Dinner:** Grilled chicken with roasted Brussels sprouts and sweet potatoes

## Day 10

- ★ **Breakfast:** Scrambled eggs with spinach and mushrooms

- ★ **Snack:** sugar-free almond milk latte

- ★ **Lunch:** Tuna salad with mixed greens and sugar-free ranch dressing

- ★ **Snack:** sugar-free coconut milk yogurt with chia seeds

- ★ **Dinner:** Grilled steak with roasted sweet potato and green beans

# Day 11

* **Breakfast:** Vegan protein smoothie with almond milk, spinach, and chia seeds

* **Snack:** raw veggies with hummus

* **Lunch:** Grilled chicken with mixed greens salad and sugar-free balsamic vinaigrette

* **Snack:** sugar-free coconut milk yogurt with mixed berries

* **Dinner:** Baked salmon with roasted asparagus and quinoa

# Day 12

* **Breakfast:** Vegan protein pancakes with sugar-free maple syrup and mixed berries

* **Snack:** A sugar-free protein bar

* **Lunch:** Turkey chili with mixed green salad

* **Snack:** Sugar-free coconut milk yogurt with sliced almonds

* **Dinner:** Grilled shrimp, zucchini noodles, and tomato sauce

# Day 13

* **Breakfast:** Vegan protein smoothie with almond milk, spinach, and chia seeds

* **Snack:** Raw veggies with guacamole

* **Lunch:** Chicken salad with mixed greens and sugar-free balsamic vinaigrette

* **Snack:** sugar-free coconut milk yogurt with mixed berries

* **Dinner:** Baked chicken with roasted broccoli and cauliflower rice

# Day 14

* **Breakfast:** Scrambled eggs with spinach and mushrooms

* **Snack:** sugar-free almond milk latte

* **Lunch:** Tuna salad with mixed greens and sugar-free ranch dressing

* **Snack:** sugar-free coconut milk yogurt with chia seeds

* **Dinner:** Grilled steak with roasted sweet potato and green beans

These meals are designed to be Candida-friendly, utilizing ingredients that are known to fight Candida overgrowth. The meal plan includes a variety of protein sources, healthy fats, and complex carbohydrates to keep you feeling full and satisfied throughout the day. The nutritional value of each meal will depend on the specific ingredients used, but all meals are designed to be low in sugar and high in fiber.

# CONCLUSION

In conclusion, embarking on a Candida cleanse journey is a powerful step towards reclaiming your health and vitality. By following the recipes in this cookbook, you have taken the first step towards a healthier, more balanced life. As you celebrate the completion of this cleanse, it's important to reflect on the positive changes you've experienced. You may have noticed increased energy, improved digestion, and a greater sense of well-being. These changes are a testament to the healing power of the foods you've consumed during this cleanse.

Moving forward, it's essential to maintain a diet that supports your overall health and well-being. By incorporating Candida-friendly recipes into your daily meals, you can continue to support a healthy balance of gut flora and promote overall wellness. Additionally, staying mindful of your food choices and their impact on your body will help you make informed decisions that support your long-term health goals.

As you close this chapter, remember that the knowledge and experience you've gained during this cleanse are valuable tools for creating a healthier future. By continuing to prioritize whole, nourishing foods and a balanced lifestyle, you can support your body's natural ability to thrive. Congratulations on completing this cleanse, and here's to a future filled with vibrant health and vitality.

Please email me at loefflerlaura753@gmail.com if you have any questions regarding this cookbook.

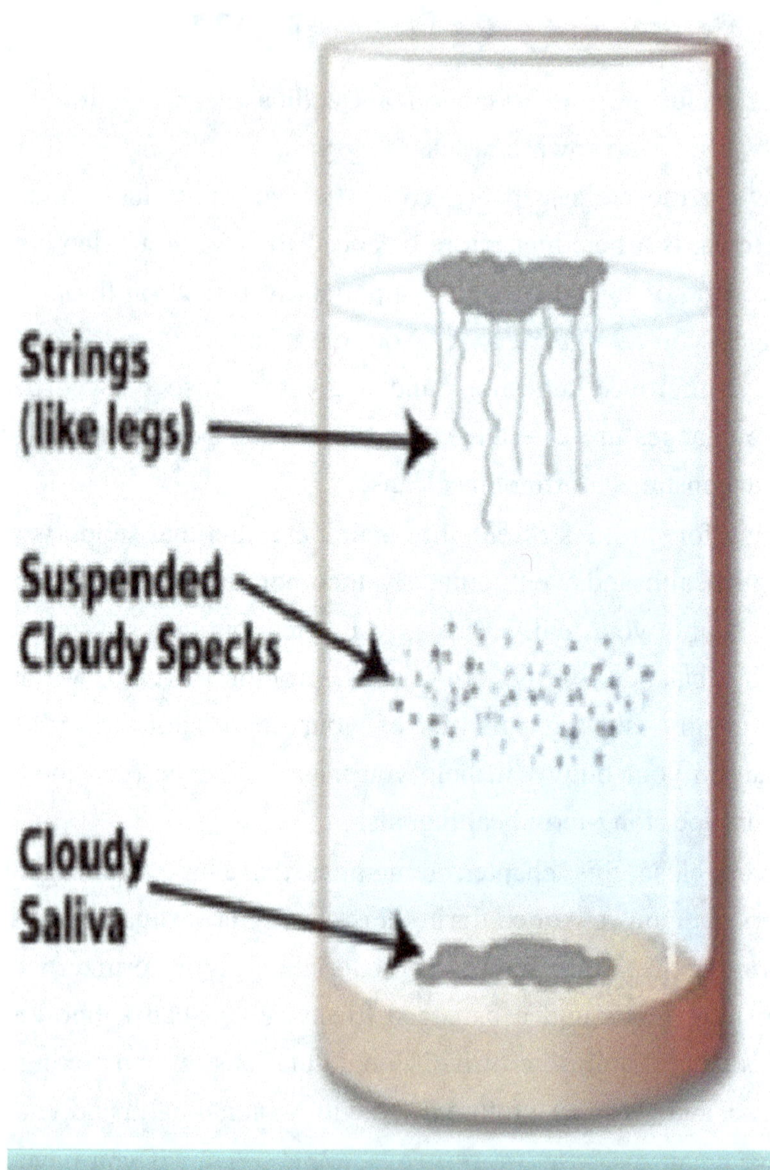

Strings
(like legs)
Suspended
Cloudy Specks
Cloudy
Saliva
CANDIDA TENTACLES

# 14 DAY MEAL PLANNER JOURNAL

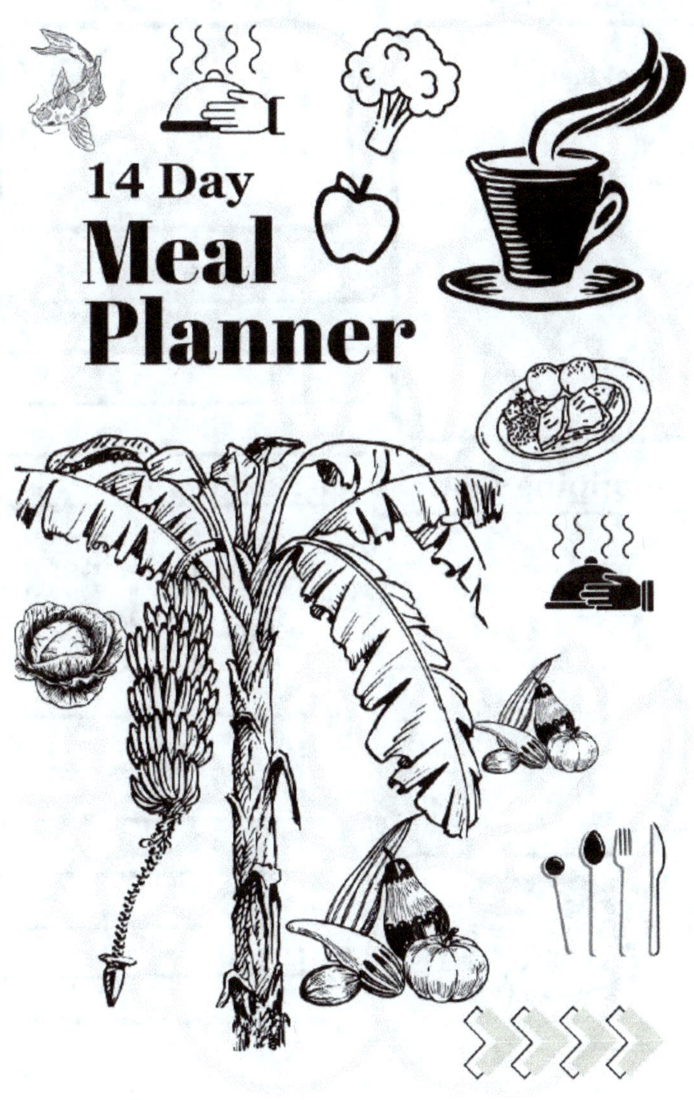

## Menu List:

**Breakfast:**

**Lunch:**

**Snacks:**

**Dinner:**

## Main Meal:

## To Do List:

## Shopping List:

TO BUY

SALAD

## Note and Tips:

**To-Do**

## Menu List:

Breakfast:

Lunch:

Snacks:

Dinner:

## Main Meal:

## To Do List:

## Shopping List:

TO BUY

SALAD

## Note and Tips:

To-Do

**Date/Day:**          **Week:**          **Water:**

## Menu List:

**Breakfast:**

**Lunch:**

**Snacks:**

**Dinner:**

## Main Meal:

## To Do List:

## Shopping List:

## Note and Tips:

To-Do

## Menu List:

**Breakfast:**

**Lunch:**

**Snacks:**

**Dinner:**

## Main Meal:

## To Do List:

## Shopping List:

TO BUY



## Note and Tips:

## Menu List:

**Breakfast:**

**Lunch:**

**Snacks:**

**Dinner:**

## Main Meal:

## To Do List:

## Shopping List:

TO BUY

SALAD

## Note and Tips:

To-Do

**Date/Day:**     **Week:**

**Water:**

## Menu List:

**Breakfast:**

**Lunch:**

**Snacks:**

**Dinner:**

## Main Meal:

## To Do List:

## Shopping List:



## Note and Tips:

**Date/Day:**          **Week:**          **Water:**

## Menu List:

**Breakfast:**

**Lunch:**

**Snacks:**

**Dinner:**

## Main Meal:

## To Do List:

## Shopping List:



## Note and Tips:

## Menu List:

Breakfast:

Lunch:

Snacks:

Dinner:

## Main Meal:

## To Do List:

## Shopping List:




## Note and Tips:

**Date/Day:**          **Week:**          **Water:**

## Menu List:

**Breakfast:**

**Lunch:**

**Snacks:**

**Dinner:**

## Main Meal:

## To Do List:

## Shopping List:

## Note and Tips:

**To-Do**

## Menu List:

Breakfast:

Lunch:

Snacks:

Dinner:

## Main Meal:

## To Do List:

## Shopping List:





## Note and Tips:

## Menu List:

Breakfast:

Lunch:

Snacks:

Dinner:

## Main Meal:

## To Do List:

## Shopping List:

## Note and Tips:

To-Do

**Date/Day:**          **Week:**

**Water:**

## Menu List:

**Breakfast:**

**Lunch:**

**Snacks:**

**Dinner:**

## Main Meal:

## To Do List:

## Shopping List:

## Note and Tips:

**To-Do**

TO BUY

SALAD

**Date/Day:**          **Week:**

**Water:**

## Menu List:

**Breakfast:**

**Lunch:**

**Snacks:**

**Dinner:**

## Main Meal:

## To Do List:

## Shopping List:





## Note and Tips:

www.ingramcontent.com/pod-product-compliance
Lightning Source LLC
Chambersburg PA
CBHW070844250726

48662CB00003B/1351